LIVING WITH
DIABETES

CANADIAN DIABETES ASSOCIATION | ASSOCIATION CANADIENNE DU DIABÈTE

LIVING WITH
DIABETES

Rosemary Walker & Jill Rodgers

Editor-in-Chief for Canada Donna Lillie

Editor, Canada Julia Roles
Project Editor, Canada Ian Whitelaw
Senior Editors Dawn Henderson, Kesta Desmond, Jill Hamilton
Senior Art Editor Catherine MacKenzie
Senior Managing Editor Martyn Page
Managing Art Editor Marianne Markham
DTP Designer Julian Dams
Production Controllers Wendy Penn, Kirsti Rippon
Production Manager Sarah Coltman
Category Publishers Mary Thompson, Corinne Roberts
Art Director Bryn Walls

Produced for Dorling Kindersley by
COOLING BROWN

First Canadian Edition, 2006

Dorling Kindersley is represented in Canada by
Tourmaline Editions Inc., 662 King Street West, Suite 304, Toronto, Ontario M5V 1M7

Every effort has been made to ensure that the information in this book is accurate. The information in this book may not be applicable in each individual case so you are therefore advised to obtain expert medical advice for specific information on personal health matters. Never disregard expert medical advice or delay in receiving advice or treatment due to information obtained from this book. The naming of any product, treatment, or organization in this book does not imply endorsement by the authors, the CDA, or publisher, nor does the omission of such names indicate disapproval. The publisher, authors, and the CDA cannot accept legal responsibility for any personal injury or other damage or loss arising from any use or misuse of the information and advice in this book.

Library and Archives Canada Cataloguing in Publication
Walker, Rosemary
    Living with diabetes : a practical guide to managing your health /
Rosemary Walker, Jill Rodgers. -- Canadian ed. / Donna Lillie, editor-in-chief.
Includes index.
ISBN-13: 978-1-55363-058-6
ISBN-10: 1-55363-058-0
    1. Diabetes--Popular works. I. Rodgers, Jill II. Lillie, Donna
III. Title.
RC660.4.W35 2006   616.4'62   C2005-903354-1

Reproduced by Colourscan, Singapore
Printed and bound by Star Standard, Singapore

06 07 08 09 10 9 8 7 6 5 4 3 2 1

Discover more at
www.dk.com

Foreword

More than 2 million Canadians have diabetes, and this number is expected to reach 3 million by the year 2010. If you or someone you know has been affected by diabetes, you are probably already aware that it is a complex disease, requiring careful adjustments of lifestyle and medication in order to maintain good health. Knowledge is the first step in managing this condition. The purpose of this book is to provide useful, practical information to help people living with diabetes.

This book has been completely edited by the Canadian Diabetes Association to reflect their *Clinical Practice Guidelines for the Prevention and Management of Diabetes in Canada*. These evidence-based guidelines consolidate the best available science from around the world concerning the prevention, diagnosis, and management of diabetes and its complications.

Once diabetes is diagnosed, living a healthy lifestyle and managing blood glucose levels to targets that will assist in the delay and prevention of both long- and short-term complications becomes a part of daily living. There has never been a more challenging or hopeful time in the diabetes world, as new therapeutics become available and new knowledge drives better care and management. The Canadian Diabetes Association encourages all Canadians affected by diabetes to learn as much as possible about the condition and the necessary regular medical assessments to ensure an optimal quality of life.

Donna Lillie
Vice President, Research & Professional Education
Canadian Diabetes Association

Contents

LIVING WITH DIABETES

CHILDREN AND TEENAGERS

POSSIBLE LONG-TERM COMPLICATIONS

What is diabetes?

Today about 200 million people worldwide have diabetes, and this number is increasing by more than 20 million each year.

If you or someone close to you has diabetes, it's important to understand as much as you can about the condition. This chapter gives an overview of diabetes, explaining how the healthy body uses glucose (sugar) and how and why a person with diabetes is unable to use glucose in this way.

There is no single cause of diabetes but there are risk factors that, in combination, increase your chances of developing the condition. These risk factors can be related to your genes, the environment, or your lifestyle. How quickly you are diagnosed with diabetes depends, in part, on the nature and severity of your symptoms.

Although diabetes has an impact on your day-to-day health, it can also have serious effects on your long-term health. If your blood glucose level is regularly elevated over a period of years, this can cause damage to your eyes, kidneys, feet, and heart, for example. This is why effective long-term management of your diabetes is so important.

Understanding diabetes

To understand diabetes, you need to know how the hormone insulin usually controls your blood glucose level and what happens inside your body when this control breaks down. There are different types of diabetes, but in each type glucose accumulates in your blood to a level that could be harmful to your health. Whether you develop diabetes, and which type you develop, is the result of a combination of inherited and environmental factors.

What is diabetes?

Diabetes is a condition in which your body cannot control the level of glucose (sugar) in your blood because your pancreas does not produce insulin, does not produce enough insulin, or your body cells are resistant to the action of insulin. Therefore, when your blood glucose level rises, the glucose cannot get into your body cells, which are therefore deprived of their usual source of energy. Your body responds by trying to eliminate excess glucose from your blood and by using fat and protein (from muscle) as alternative sources of energy. This disrupts your bodily processes and can cause some of the symptoms of diabetes (see pp.18–19).

How the healthy body uses glucose

When you eat carbohydrate foods such as bread, rice, potatoes, cereals, or sugar, they are broken down into glucose during digestion. Glucose moves from the intestines into the bloodstream and then enters the body's cells, where it is burned as fuel—it powers your entire body, from the muscles to the brain, and is the body's primary source of energy. Glucose is also stored in the liver and muscles in the form of glycogen.

Two of the main hormones that control blood glucose are insulin and glucagon. Both are produced in the pancreas, a gland that lies behind the stomach. There are clusters of cells in the pancreas called the islets of Langerhans; within these are two types of hormone-producing cells, alpha and beta cells: alpha cells produce glucagon; beta cells produce insulin.

There is a constant background level of insulin in your body but when your blood glucose level rises—after eating, for example—extra insulin is released by your beta cells. Insulin acts like a key, unlocking

OBESITY AND DIABETES
There is growing recognition
that the increase in type 2
diabetes in the West is
associated with obesity
and a sedentary lifestyle.

body cells so that glucose can enter.
When your blood glucose level
falls—after a period without food, for
example—your alpha cells release
more glucagon, which converts
glycogen in your liver back to glucose.
This enters your bloodstream and
your blood glucose level rises again.
Insulin and glucagon work together
constantly in this way to ensure that
your blood glucose level stays within
a close range of 4–7 millimoles of
glucose per liter (mmol/L) of blood.
As a result, whether you have eaten a
lot of carbohydrate or a little, your
body has the constant supply of
energy it needs to work properly.

What goes wrong in diabetes?

When you have diabetes, the finely
tuned system that regulates blood
glucose fails because you don't
produce insulin, or you don't produce
enough of it, or your body is resistant

THE HEALTHY BODY'S RESPONSE TO GLUCOSE

Glucose is the body's primary energy source. The quantity of
glucose in your blood is carefully regulated by two pancreatic
hormones, insulin and glucagon. As a result, despite variations in
the amount of carbohydrate you eat, your body has a constant
supply of glucose from which to produce energy.

Glucose enters bloodstream after eating and drinking

Blood glucose level rises

Glucagon converts glycogen (from liver) to glucose, which enters blood

Pancreas produces insulin

Pancreas produces glucagon

Insulin enables cells to take in glucose

Blood glucose level falls

Cells "burn" glucose to produce energy; liver cells convert glucose to glycogen to insulin. As a result, glucose cannot pass into your cells to be burned for energy, and it builds up in the blood. This leads to an abnormally high blood glucose level.

A high blood glucose level

When you have an elevated blood glucose level you may experience symptoms such as urinating large amounts and excessive thirst. This is because your body removes excess glucose by filtering it through your kidneys and into your urine (the thirst is a result of dehydration). Also, because your body cannot use glucose properly for energy, it obtains energy by breaking down your muscle and fat stores. This can cause weight loss and, in the case of rapid fat breakdown, the buildup of toxic chemicals in your blood. Unfortunately, an elevated blood glucose level does not always produce symptoms, and only a blood glucose test (see pp.70–73) can tell you that it is high. A blood glucose level that is consistently high over a period of years can damage the body's

tissues, leading to complications involving your eyes, kidneys, feet, heart, blood vessels, and nerves.

Types of diabetes

There are two main types of diabetes: type 1 and type 2, the latter being the most common. Although they are both types of diabetes, type 1 and type 2 are very different conditions. There are also other types of diabetes that affect a minority of people: gestational diabetes, maturity onset diabetes of the young (MODY), and rarer forms that are related to infections, medications, and pancreas disease or damage.

Type 1 diabetes

Previously known as "juvenile onset" or "insulin-dependent" diabetes, type 1 affects fewer than 1 in 5 people with diabetes. It usually appears during childhood, adolescence, or early adulthood, but can appear at any age. If you have type 1 diabetes, you don't produce any insulin because the beta

THE PANCREAS
Lying deep within the abdomen and behind the stomach, the pancreas is a gland that secretes all the body's insulin—one of the hormones that regulates the level of glucose in the blood. The cells in the pancreas that manufacture and release insulin are called beta cells and are found in the islets of Langerhans.

Liver

Stomach

Pancreas

Intestine

White spaces show the breakdown of the islets of Langerhans and destruction of beta cells within them

Islets of Langerhans

Tissue from a healthy pancreas

Tissue from the pancreas of a person with type 1 diabetes

TYPE 1 DIABETES—YOUR BODY'S RESPONSE TO GLUCOSE

If you have type 1 diabetes, your pancreas does not produce any insulin. This means that your blood glucose level rises unchecked and your body is deprived of its primary energy source. This results in fatigue, lack of energy, frequent urination, dehydration, thirst, and weight loss. To compensate for the lack of glucose, your body breaks down fat and protein (from muscle) as an alternative energy source. This can lead to a potentially life-threatening condition called diabetic ketoacidosis. Your pancreas still produces glucagon, another pancreatic hormone involved in blood glucose control.

> If you have type 1 diabetes, you don't produce any insulin because the beta cells in your pancreas have been destroyed.

The rising incidence of obesity associated with a sedentary Western lifestyle may trigger type 2 diabetes.

TYPE 2 DIABETES—YOUR BODY'S RESPONSE TO GLUCOSE

If you have type 2 diabetes, your body cells are resistant to the action of insulin and/or your pancreas produces decreasing amounts of insulin. As a result, your blood glucose level becomes progressively higher over time and your body cells receive an inadequate supply of glucose—your body's primary energy source. This may result in a range of symptoms including fatigue, lack of energy, frequent urination, thirst, and gradual weight loss. To make up for insufficient glucose, your body may break down fat and protein (from muscle) as additional energy sources. Since your pancreas still produces some insulin, however, you are highly unlikely to develop diabetic ketoacidosis, because your body doesn't become entirely dependent on fat as an energy source (as in type 1 diabetes).

Glucose enters bloodstream after eating and drinking

Blood glucose level rises

Cells resistant to insulin and/or pancreas cannot produce enough insulin

Cells can only take in small amounts of glucose from blood

Blood glucose level remains high

With limited glucose, cells have reduced energy

Kidneys produce extra urine to remove glucose from blood

Small amounts of fat may be broken down as alternative source of energy

Symptoms: fatigue, lack of energy

Symptoms: passing a lot of urine, leading to dehydration and thirst; urinary tract infections; blurred vision

Symptom: gradual weight loss; can also cause damage to blood vessels and general infections

If blood glucose rises very high, there is a risk of extreme dehydration leading to loss of consciousness cells in your pancreas have been destroyed. In most cases, this is the result of an autoimmune response in which your immune system mistakenly treats your beta cells as foreign bodies and attacks them. This response may be triggered by a viral infection. Although type 1 seems to develop suddenly, the destruction of beta cells can start months or years earlier. It is not until your beta cells are functioning at less than 10 percent of their capacity that diabetes symptoms appear.

Type 1 diabetes is treated with insulin, given by injection or via a pump (see pp.82–101). You cannot take insulin in tablet form because it would be destroyed during digestion.

Type 2 diabetes

Previously known as "maturity-onset" or "non-insulin-dependent" diabetes, type 2 diabetes affects 4 in 5 people with diabetes and tends to develop after the age of 40. The rising incidence of obesity associated with a sedentary Western lifestyle may trigger type 2 diabetes. It is also becoming increasingly common for children and teenagers to develop type 2 diabetes for this reason.

If you have type 2 diabetes, you produce insulin, but in insufficient amounts and/or your body cells are resistant to the action of insulin. Initially, your pancreas responds to insulin resistance by producing more insulin but, over time, your pancreas cannot keep up with your body's demand for insulin—this is why the treatment of type 2 diabetes changes over time. At first, losing weight, healthier eating, and physical activity may keep your blood glucose level well controlled, sometimes for years. When necessary, you are prescribed pills that increase the amount of insulin in your blood, improve your insulin's function, or change the rate at which carbohydrate is broken down during digestion. Eventually, you will probably need insulin injections, too.

COMPARING TYPE 1 AND TYPE 2 DIABETES

Although they share some of the same symptoms, type 1 and type 2 diabetes are really separate conditions, and there are separate causes and treatments for each.

TYPE 1 DIABETES	TYPE 2 DIABETES
Usually starts in childhood or early adulthood; rarely develops after age 40.	Usually starts in adulthood, often after age 40, but increasingly common at a younger age.
The body doesn't produce insulin because the insulin-producing beta cells in the pancreas have been destroyed.	The body produces insulin, but it is resistant to its action. Over time, insulin production progressively declines.
People affected are usually underweight or normal weight.	People affected are usually overweight.
People affected need insulin treatment, as well as care with eating and physical activity.	People affected need care with healthy eating, physical activity, and pill and insulin treatment.
Frequent urination, excessive thirst, weight loss, and fatigue can come on quickly and be severe.	Frequent urination, excessive thirst, weight loss, fatigue, and blurred vision may be gradual, mild, or absent.
Diagnosis is usually rapid— within days or weeks of the development of symptoms.	Diabetes may not be diagnosed for several years.
Children of people with type 1 diabetes have a 1–6 percent chance of developing type 1 diabetes.	Children of people with type 2 diabetes have a 14 percent chance of developing type 2 diabetes.
Cannot be prevented.	Risk reduced by weight reduction and regular physical activity.

Gestational diabetes

This type of diabetes may develop around the 28th week (6th month) of pregnancy and is the only temporary form of diabetes. For more about gestational diabetes, see pp.144–145.

Maturity onset diabetes of the young (MODY)

This is a rare type of diabetes that affects about 1 in 100 people with diabetes. MODY usually becomes apparent in the teens or 20s. It is similar to type 2 diabetes but develops only in people with specific genes that cause a defect in the way the insulin-producing cells in the pancreas work. This leads to underproduction of insulin. MODY can be confirmed by genetic testing.

Treatment—as with type 2 diabetes—usually focuses on healthy eating and physical activity first, then treatment with pills and/or insulin if necessary.

GESTATIONAL DIABETES
The hormonal changes of pregnancy can lead to insulin resistance and temporary diabetes in some women. Gestational diabetes usually disappears when pregnancy is over but can reappear in future pregnancies and greatly increases a woman's risk of developing type 2 diabetes in later life.

Why does diabetes develop?

Diabetes has no single cause, but may be caused by a combination of any of the following inherited and environmental factors.

■ **GENES** If you have the specific genes for type 1 diabetes, you may develop it at some point in your life, although this is not inevitable. If you don't have the genes for type 1 diabetes, you will not develop it (unless your pancreas is removed). In type 2 diabetes there is no specific genetic pattern, but your chances of developing it increase if members of your family have the condition (see opposite). There are also certain genetic syndromes that, although rare, can increase your risk of developing diabetes, the most common being Down syndrome, which can lead to type 2 diabetes.

■ **WEIGHT** If you are overweight, you have an increased risk of developing type 2 diabetes because your body cells may become resistant to insulin. Obesity, defined as weighing 20 percent more than your ideal body weight (see p.46), further increases your risk. Being overweight does not increase your risk of type 1 diabetes.

■ **BODY SHAPE** If you carry excess weight around your waist, you have a higher risk of developing type 2 diabetes (but not type 1 diabetes) than if you carry excess weight on your hips and thighs (see p.45).

■ **ETHNIC BACKGROUND** If you are of African, Latin American, Aboriginal, or Asian descent, you have five times more chance of developing type 2 diabetes than people of Caucasian origin (but you are no more likely to develop type 1 diabetes).

■ **PREGNANCY** When you are pregnant your body increases its blood glucose level in order to cope with the demands of a growing baby; therefore more insulin is needed. If your body can't produce enough insulin for your needs and those of the fetus, your blood glucose level remains high and gestational diabetes is diagnosed.

■ **MEDICATIONS** Some medicines can raise your blood glucose level or prevent insulin from working properly. If you take any of these medicines, you have a higher chance of developing type 2 diabetes.

• Steroids, such as prednisone and cortisone, which are used to treat inflammatory conditions.

• Thiazide diuretics, such as hydrochlorthiazide, which are used to remove excess fluid from the body.

• Beta-blockers, such as propranolol, which are used to treat hypertension (high blood pressure).

• Immunosuppressants, such as cyclosporine, which are used to prevent rejection of organs, following a transplant.

■ **VIRAL INFECTIONS** Specific infections, which may have occurred up to two years earlier, may trigger type 1 diabetes if you are genetically predisposed to it. A virus can set off an abnormal reaction in which your immune system destroys the insulin-producing cells in your pancreas. Viral infections do not trigger type 2 diabetes.

■ **DAMAGE TO THE PANCREAS** The following conditions may lead to the development of diabetes:

• Pancreatitis (an inflammation of the pancreas).

• Cystic fibrosis (a genetic condition that causes body secretions to be abnormally thick).

• Hemochromatosis (a buildup of excess iron that gradually damages the insulin-producing cells).

• Removal of the pancreas. If your pancreas is removed due to disease, such as cancer, or an accident, type 1 diabetes develops because you are no longer able to produce insulin.

■ **HORMONAL DISORDERS** If your body overproduces hormones that oppose the action of insulin, your risk of developing type 2 diabetes increases. The main hormonal disorders linked with diabetes are Cushing disease, in which the adrenal glands produce excess steroid hormones, and acromegaly, in which the pituitary gland overproduces growth hormone.

CHANCES OF INHERITING DIABETES

Having diabetes in your family increases the risk of you developing it too. This table shows your increased risk of developing diabetes, depending on which of your close relatives has diabetes.

FAMILY MEMBER	YOUR INCREASED RISK
Mother with type 1	1–2%
Mother with type 2	14%
Father with type 1	3–6%
Father with type 2	14%
Both parents with type 1	30%
Both parents with type 2	75%
Sibling with type 1	6%
Sibling with type 2	15–25%
Identical twin with type 1	30%
Identical twin with type 2	50–100%
No relatives with diabetes	No increased risk

If you carry excess weight around your waist, you have a higher risk of developing type 2 diabetes.

Symptoms and diagnosis

The symptoms of both types of diabetes are similar, but they tend to be more acute at diagnosis in type 1, and develop more gradually—even over many years—in type 2. If you think you may have diabetes, see your doctor as soon as possible. The condition is diagnosed with one or more blood tests. If these tests confirm that you have diabetes, you will have other tests to assess your health and check for any signs of the long-term complications of diabetes.

Recognizing diabetes

It is more common to notice the symptoms of a high blood glucose level if you have type 1 diabetes, because the absence of insulin has a dramatic effect on your body. If you have type 2 diabetes, you still produce some insulin, so your symptoms may be less severe—you may even attribute them to growing older. For example, you may think it's normal to feel tired, or to get up at night to urinate. Occasionally with type 2, there are no symptoms at all and diabetes may not even be suspected until you have a routine medical or eye test that reveals early signs of long-term complications. The following are all symptoms of diabetes.

■ **URINATING FREQUENTLY** When your blood glucose level reaches a certain level, your kidneys filter excess glucose out of your blood. To expel it from your body, more urine is produced; therefore you need to urinate more often. You may not notice this during the day, but you may wake up two or three times a night to urinate.

■ **DRY MOUTH, EXCESSIVE THIRST** Since you are urinating frequently you become dehydrated, which causes thirst and a dry mouth. Quenching your thirst with sugary drinks can aggravate the problem by raising your blood glucose even higher, so drink sugar-free drinks.

■ **LACK OF ENERGY** You may feel tired all the time, find it difficult to carry out

My experience

"I couldn't stop urinating and I had this incredible thirst. One day I was so thirsty that I found myself drinking from the cold-water faucet while I sat on the toilet." JULIE

COMMENT Frequent urination and intense thirst are two symptoms of diabetes. When blood glucose reaches 10 millimoles per liter, excess glucose is passed out in the urine. Large amounts of water (to dilute the glucose) are lost, causing dehydration and thirst.

day-to-day activities, and still feel tired even if you rest or sleep more than usual. This is because some or all of the glucose in your blood cannot enter your body cells to give you energy.

■ **WEIGHT LOSS** When your body cannot use glucose, it starts to break down its fat and muscle stores for energy instead. As a result you may lose weight. Weight loss is more common and rapid in type 1 than type 2 diabetes. In type 2, weight loss may happen very slowly or not at all.

If you are overweight, you may be pleased to lose weight in such an effortless way. This isn't healthy, however, and, as soon as your diabetes is under control, you should expect to regain the weight that you have lost.

■ **BLURRED VISION** When your blood glucose level is high, the lenses of your eyes absorb glucose and water. This makes them swell, which causes blurred vision.

■ **FRUITY-SMELLING BREATH** This is a late symptom of type 1 diabetes and indicates a dangerously high blood glucose level. When your body breaks down fat for energy it produces toxic by-products called ketones. If your breath has a fruity smell (the smell is often said to be similar to that of nail polish remover), this is a sign that your body is trying to expel ketones through your lungs. If you also develop any of the following symptoms—nausea, vomiting, and/or abdominal pain—you may need urgent hospital treatment for ketoacidosis (diabetic coma), which although rare, can be extremely dangerous (see p.113).

■ **YEAST AND CYSTITIS** The presence of glucose in your urine provides a good environment for bacteria and germs to grow in large amounts, making yeast infections and cystitis more likely.

Fruity-smelling breath is a late symptom of type 1 diabetes and indicates a dangerously high blood glucose level.

MEDICAL TESTS USED IN THE DIAGNOSIS AND MANAGEMENT OF DIABETES

Although urine and fingerprick tests can reveal a higher than normal blood glucose level, you need one or more of three laboratory blood tests to diagnose diabetes: the random or fasting blood glucose test and, if necessary, the oral glucose tolerance test. Your results are assessed with your symptoms. If you don't have symptoms but diabetes is suspected, you need a repeat blood test carried out on a different day.

HOW THE TEST IS CARRIED OUT	WHAT THE RESULTS MEAN

Urine test

A health professional tests a sample of your urine using a dipstick that changes color according to the amount of glucose present. The dipstick is then compared with a color chart. A result is obtained within 1 minute.

The presence or absence of glucose in urine does not necessarily indicate or discount diabetes. If your urine contains glucose, or you have symptoms but no glucose, you will be referred for further blood tests.

Fingerprick test

A health professional uses a device to prick the side of your fingertip and puts a drop of blood from your finger onto a testing strip. This strip is then inserted in a blood glucose meter in the laboratory to be analyzed. A result is obtained within 1 minute.

A healthy blood glucose level is within the range of 4.0–6.1 millimoles per liter (mmol/L). If your test result is higher than 6.1 mmol/L, your health professional will ask you to have further blood tests. A fingerprick test by itself is not enough to diagnose diabetes.

Fasting blood glucose test

You do not eat or drink overnight; in the morning your health professional takes a blood sample from your arm. The sample is sent to a laboratory for analysis. Your health professional receives the results within a week.

If you have symptoms and a test result higher than 6.9 millimoles of glucose per liter, you have diabetes. If you have no symptoms, or the result is less and you have symptoms, you may repeat the test or take an oral glucose tolerance test.

Random blood glucose test

Your health professional takes a blood sample from your arm to send to a laboratory for analysis. This sample can be taken regardless of whether you have eaten. Your health professional receives the results within a week.

If you have symptoms and a test result higher than 11.1 millimoles of glucose per liter, diabetes is diagnosed. If you have no symptoms, or the result is less, you may repeat the test while fasting or take an oral glucose tolerance test.

Oral glucose tolerance test

You do not eat or drink overnight; in the morning your health professional takes a blood sample from your arm before and 2 hours after you have a drink containing some glucose. The samples are sent for analysis. Your health professional usually receives the results in a week.

If your fasting level is above 6.9 millimoles of glucose per liter (mmol/L) and/or your 2-hour test result is above 11.1 mmol/L, diabetes is diagnosed, whether or not you have symptoms. This test is used if other tests are inconclusive and to diagnose gestational diabetes.

Diagnosing diabetes

Diabetes must be diagnosed on the basis of a blood test in which a blood sample is analyzed in a laboratory (see opposite). type 1 diabetes is likely to be diagnosed more quickly than type 2, because the symptoms usually develop rapidly and are more severe. type 2 diabetes is sometimes suspected when you are showing early signs of complications. For example, abnormal changes at the back of your eye may be noticed at a routine eye examination.

Your diabetes will be diagnosed by one or more of three blood tests: a random blood glucose test, a fasting blood glucose test, and an oral glucose tolerance test. Tests such as fingerprick and urine tests are not sufficient to confirm or discount the presence of diabetes (see opposite). If your fasting blood glucose level is 6.1–6.9 millimoles per liter, your blood glucose is not normal, but not high enough for diabetes to be diagnosed. Your health professional will explain what your test results mean and the implications they have for you.

Medical tests after diagnosis

One of the main aims of diabetes care is to prevent long-term complications.Within about three months of diagnosis, you will be offered the following routine tests to check your general health too and look for signs that any complications may be developing. Your test results form the starting point for your yearly checkup, known as your annual

review (see p.26). If any problems are discovered, you will be referred for the appropriate treatment.

■ **HEIGHT, WEIGHT, AND BODY MASS INDEX** Your body mass index (BMI) is calculated (see p.46). Your BMI shows whether you are overweight for your height.

■ **BLOOD PRESSURE** Hypertension (high blood pressure) is especially common in people with type 2 diabetes. If your blood pressure is high over a period of time, medication to lower it will be prescribed.

■ **FOOT EXAMINATION** A health professional checks your foot circulation and nerve supply and teaches you how to look after your own feet (see pp.128–130).

■ **EYE EXAMINATION** The retina at the back of your eye is checked for damaged blood vessels using either an instrument known as an ophthalmoscope or an eye camera.

■ **OTHER TESTS** Blood tests are done to check kidney, liver, and thyroid function, as well as blood fat levels. An A1C test assesses your glucose level over the previous six to eight weeks (see p.23). Your urine is tested for protein (a possible sign of early kidney damage; see pp.196–199).

Type 1 diabetes is likely to be diagnosed more quickly than type 2 because the symptoms usually develop rapidly and are more severe.

Looking after your diabetes

If you look after yourself and your diabetes, you can continue to live life to the full. Regularly testing your blood glucose level, eating and drinking healthily, engaging in plenty of physical activity, and taking your pills and/or insulin injections all help you control your blood glucose level effectively. Good blood glucose control is vital to reduce your risk of developing long-term complications, and your health professional works with you to achieve this.

Monitoring blood glucose

When you have diabetes, your body cannot control your blood glucose level in the usual way. The key to caring for your diabetes is to keep your blood glucose level within the recommended range of 4–7 millimoles per liter (mmol/L). Monitoring your blood glucose level regularly and adjusting your treatment accordingly will help you achieve this. This is critical to prevent long-term complications (see pp.26–27).

My experience

"The more you know about diabetes, the better you can control it and the more flexible you can be. That message has transformed my life." JOE

COMMENT Learning as much as you can about diabetes can help you fit it into your life. Also, blood glucose monitoring helps you learn about how different situations affect your blood glucose level. Your test results enable you to make informed decisions about how to control your diabetes.

Home testing

Measuring your own blood glucose is easier and more accurate than ever before. There is a wide range of testing equipment available, from basic blood testing strips to sophisticated electronic meters with computer download facilities that allow you to analyze the results (see pp.67–70).

When and how often you test your blood glucose largely depends on your treatment, the food you eat, and your physical activity. The aim is to find a time and frequency that suits you and gives you the information you need to control your diabetes effectively. For a step-by-step guide to blood glucose testing, see pp.62–75.

Whatever type of diabetes you have, the recommended blood glucose level to aim for is 4–7 mmol/L. This range is close enough to the range of people who do not have diabetes to reduce the risk of possible long-term complications.

The A1C test

Although testing your blood glucose level at home is a key part of diabetes care there is another type of blood glucose test, the A1C test, which is carried out by a health professional every three months. The difference between this and your home tests is that the A1C test gives an overall measure of your blood glucose level for the previous six to eight weeks, while the home tests give day-to-day readings of your blood glucose level. A1C results are given as a percentage—the closer they are to 7 percent (or below) the better.

Controlling blood glucose

Keeping your blood glucose level well controlled is one of the most effective ways to prevent long-term complications and keep you feeling well. Good control means that most

Q What does it mean if my A1C result is above 7 percent?

A It means that you should discuss your diabetes management with your health professional. Even a result of 7.5 percent is considered unsatisfactory control of diabetes. For every 1 percent rise in your A1C result, there is a 30 percent increase in the likelihood of developing complications that affect your blood vessels and nerves; therefore, being strict about a 7 percent result is important.

of your home blood glucose test results fall within the range of 4–7 mmol/L, and your A1C result will be close to 7 percent. The four main factors that affect your blood glucose control are food and drink you consume, your physical activity, type 2 pills, and insulin injections. When your blood glucose level is poorly controlled you will experience hypoglycemia (low blood glucose) or hyperglycemia (high blood glucose).

Good control means that most of your home blood test results fall within the range of 4–7 millimoles per liter.

Practical tips

KEEPING YOUR BLOOD GLUCOSE CONTROLLED

- Eat regular, healthy meals to avoid major fluctuations in your blood glucose level.
- Stay physically active to help your insulin work more efficiently.
- Maintain your weight within the recommended range—not only to avoid needing large amounts of insulin but also to reduce your risk of heart disease.
- Take any diabetes pills or insulin you have been prescribed every day.
- Monitor your blood glucose level closely and learn to adjust your treatment to the results.

If your blood glucose level gets very low, less glucose reaches your brain, making concentration difficult.

■ **FOOD AND DRINK** Eating regular meals based on carbohydrates throughout the day helps you avoid major fluctuations in your blood glucose level. If you have type 2 diabetes, paying attention to what you eat combined with physical activity may be enough to keep your blood glucose well controlled for several years. If you take pills and/or inject insulin, you may sometimes need to alter your eating pattern to suit the timing or dose of your treatment. (For more information on healthy eating and drinking, see pp.30–43.)

■ **PHYSICAL ACTIVITY** Keeping physically active helps you control your blood glucose level by improving your body's sensitivity to insulin. Regular activity helps to lower your blood glucose level and keep it better controlled in the long term. If you take pills or inject insulin, you need to be aware that physical activity can reduce your blood glucose level in a short time. You may need to alter your treatment accordingly. (For more information on this and on physical activity, see pp.52–59.)

■ **PILLS** You may need to take pills to control your blood glucose level if you have type 2 diabetes. Pills work by increasing the amount of insulin you produce, by helping body cells use insulin more effectively, or by slowing down carbohydrate digestion. You and your health professional can discuss which pills are likely to best control your diabetes. (For more information on tablets, see pp.76–81.)

■ **INSULIN INJECTIONS** If you have type 1 diabetes, insulin injections are used to control your blood glucose level; if you have type 2, you too may need them. There are various types of insulin, which are active for different lengths of time: some act within 5 minutes and wear off within 4 hours; others keep working for 24 hours or longer. You and your health professional decide which type is best for you (see pp.82–101).

Hypoglycemia

If you take insulin or insulin-stimulating pills, your blood glucose level may sometimes fall below 4 mmol/L. This condition is known as hypoglycemia, or having low blood glucose. Possible reasons include:

- Taking too high a dose of diabetes medication, or the wrong type of medication for you.
- Being more active than usual.
- Missing or delaying meals.
- Drinking too much alcohol without compensating with food.
- Taking insulin-stimulating pills with other drugs, such as co-trimoxazole, trimethoprim (antibacterials), monoamine oxidase inhibitors (MAOI, a type of antidepressant), and ranitidine (an antiulcer drug).
- Conditions, such as underactive thyroid or reduced kidney function, which interfere with the metabolism or excretion of insulin or pills.

The main symptoms of low blood sugar are feeling shaky, sweaty, hungry, and getting pins and needles in your lips, but the symptoms vary from person to person. If your blood glucose level gets very low (below 2.8 mmol/L), less glucose reaches your brain, making concentration difficult. People may notice that you are acting strangely. For example, you might struggle to carry out a simple task or your speech might be slurred.

If you feel a low blood sugar coming on, you need to eat or drink something that quickly raises your blood glucose level, such as glucose pills, a glucose drink, or sugar cubes. If you are confused because your blood glucose is very low, you may need other people's help to take something. This is why it is advisable to tell friends and colleagues that you have diabetes. If your low blood sugar is not treated, you may lose consciousness. (For more about low blood glucose levels, see pp.102–109).

Hyperglycemia

A high level of glucose in your blood is referred to as hyperglycemia. If your blood glucose level rises above the recommended 7 mmol/L but is lower than 10 mmol/L you are likely to still feel well. Above this level, however, the symptoms of hyperglycemia start to appear. Although mild and temporary hyperglycemia won't damage your body, a high blood glucose level over months or years can lead to long-term complications of diabetes. Reasons for hyperglycemia include:

• Not taking enough medication to lower your blood glucose level, either because you are on too low a dose

> **My experience**
>
> *"There's a tension between knowing I must look after my diabetes and feeling determined not to let it stop me from doing anything I want."* JOE
>
> **COMMENT** If you feel that diabetes dominates your life and prevents you from doing things, you might be less motivated to manage your condition effectively. Talk to your health professional about ways to integrate your treatment into your daily routine.

or because you haven't been able to take it regularly.
• Being less active than usual.
• Eating very large meals or lots of high-sugar foods.
• Being ill.

The symptoms of hyperglycemia include frequent urination, intense thirst, fatigue, and infections, such as yeast and cystitis—the same symptoms that may have prompted you to seek treatment before you were diagnosed with diabetes. If your blood glucose level continues to rise and you have type 1 diabetes, you may develop diabetic ketoacidosis (see p.113); if you have type 2 diabetes, you may develop excessive dehydration, which may lead to coma, known as a non-ketotic hyperosmolar state (see p.113). Both require hospital treatment. For more about hyperglycemia, see pp.110–113.

If you frequently have a low or high blood glucose level or swing between the two, the type, quantity, or timing of your medication, physical activity, or eating may have to be changed. Your health professional can discuss causes of hypoglycemia and hyperglycemia and suggest appropriate action.

Myth OR TRUTH?

MYTH
If I feel well, my blood glucose level must be well controlled.

TRUTH
You can feel well and still have a high blood glucose level, particularly if your body has become used to it being high—not everyone has symptoms. The best way to know your blood glucose level is to test regularly.

Working with your health professional

Treatment and care for your diabetes are individually tailored to you, based on the type of diabetes you have and how well controlled your blood glucose level and other aspects of your health are. One of the most important aspects of your medical care is your annual diabetes review.

The annual review

At your annual review, your health professional assesses how well your blood glucose level is controlled and checks for any signs of the long-term complications of diabetes. You have the same routine tests that were carried out shortly after your diagnosis (see p.21). Tests for long-term complications are described in detail on pp.186–215.

It is important to recognize that your annual review should be an exchange of information and it's fine to offer your own ideas about diabetes management (see pp.148–151). Your health professional can offer both medical and psychological help and can:

- Give you information about your type of diabetes.
- Explain how your treatment works and whether you need any changes in your treatment.
- Listen and support you if you are finding it difficult to stay motivated about managing your diabetes.
- Discuss the implications of your diabetes on your work, family, and social life, and help you work out how to overcome potential problems.
- Provide information about how often you need appointments with a health professional and how you can get in touch between visits.
- Explain which other health professionals you might need to see and why.
- Ensure that you have a written record of plans made during your visit.

The Canadian Diabetes Association recommends that you see your diabetes health professional about every three months. This may be necessary to deal with a high or low blood glucose level, to monitor changes in your treatment, or to review other aspects of your care.

Long-term complications

The complications of diabetes can cause damage slowly over a period of years without any indication that they are doing so. Complications are

ANNUAL REVIEW
In addition to assessing your blood glucose level and general health, your annual review gives you the opportunity to discuss any day-to-day problems you might have with managing your diabetes.

largely caused by a consistently high blood glucose level, which slowly damages your blood circulation and nerves over years. If you have type 1 diabetes, you are unlikely to develop any complications within the first 10 years of diagnosis. The length of time before complications develop in type 2 varies. Because type 2 diabetes can go unnoticed for many years, you may have complications at the time you are diagnosed. (For more information on long-term complications, see pp.148–151.)

Types of long-term complication

Having diabetes makes you more susceptible to a number of health conditions such as:

■ **DEPRESSION** Day-to-day pressures of living with diabetes (and anticipating possible long-term complications) may have psychological effects (see pp.186–189).

■ **EYE CONDITIONS** Damage can occur to the vessels that supply blood to the retina, at the back of your eye, leading to impaired vision. Cataracts are also more common when you have diabetes (see pp.190–195).

■ **KIDNEY CONDITIONS** Gradual damage to the kidneys' filtering system may eventually lead to kidney failure (see pp.196–199).

■ **FOOT CONDITIONS** Poor circulation and damage to nerves can lead to a loss of sensation in your feet and problems such as ulcers, damage to the bones of the foot, and even gangrene (see pp.200–205).

My experience

"I am frightened about long-term complications —it's the unknown—but my annual checkups give me an objective view of my diabetes." STUART

COMMENT The key to preventing long-term complications is to make sure that your blood glucose level is well controlled as much of the time as possible. At your annual review you are checked for signs of long-term complications and are referred for treatment if necessary.

■ **CARDIOVASCULAR CONDITIONS** Conditions include high blood pressure, hyperlipidemia, coronary artery disease, stroke, and peripheral vascular disease (see pp.206–211).

■ **OTHER CONDITIONS** Injecting can cause skin conditions, and damage to the nervous and circulatory systems can cause erectile dysfunction and autonomic neuropathy (see pp.212–215).

Preventing complications

Because the long-term complications of diabetes are largely caused by too much glucose in your blood over a long period of time, any improvement you make in controlling blood glucose is beneficial. Eating a healthy diet, being physically active, losing weight if you need to, and stopping smoking, also greatly reduce your risk of developing complications. It is also important to check your feet daily (see pp.128–130) and seek help if you notice any injuries or abnormalities. Other actions that improve your control are taking your daily pills and/or insulin correctly, having an annual review, and keeping your knowledge of diabetes up to date.

Complications of diabetes can cause damage slowly over a period of years without any sign that they are doing so.

Food, drink, and physical activity

The guidelines for healthy eating and drinking and being active apply to everyone, but are especially important if you have diabetes. If you have type 2 diabetes, you may be able to manage your condition effectively with food, drink, and physical activity. If you take insulin or pills for your diabetes, you can also influence your blood glucose level by using the information in this chapter.

There are compelling health reasons for taking steps to prevent weight gain and obesity when you have diabetes. If you are overweight, losing weight can improve how well your blood glucose level is controlled.

Becoming more active can also help you lose weight. In addition, regular physical activity has benefits for your overall health and well-being, as well as your diabetes. By being aware of the impact that physical activity has on your blood glucose level, you will be able to adjust your diabetes treatment if necessary.

Healthy eating and drinking

Having diabetes is about making healthy eating choices whenever you can, eating regularly (or at the right times to balance the effects of any pills and/or insulin you take) and being aware of the effects of drinking alcohol. Knowing what's in your food—carbohydrates, protein, fat, vitamins, minerals, and fiber—enables you to make choices that help control your blood glucose level. Whether you cook at home or eat out, there are many ways to enjoy food and care for your diabetes.

You need to eat carbohydrate-containing foods because they are your body's main source of energy, but choosing those that have less immediate effect on blood glucose helps your body deal with them.

Healthy eating principles

The principles of healthy eating for people with diabetes are the same as those for everyone else. No foods are banned—but some should be eaten less often. Sometimes you don't have a choice about what food is available, but generally you can adapt recipes and meals so that you can enjoy food while eating healthily. The principles of healthy eating are as follows:
- Eat meals that contain carbohydrate at regular times.
- Eat more high-fiber foods, including fruit and vegetables (at least 5 portions per day).
- Choose whole-grain foods if possible.
- Cut down on fat.
- Eat red meat in moderation.
- Limit added sugar/sugary foods.
- Reduce your salt intake.
- Keep your alcohol consumption to the recommended limits.

Food and diabetes

When you have diabetes, your body is unable to use foods that contain carbohydrate in the usual way. All foods containing carbohydrate are broken down into glucose. You need insulin in order to allow glucose into your cells for energy now, as well as to store some glucose in your liver for energy later. Because you either have less insulin available or your insulin is not working effectively, your blood glucose level will rise when you eat carbohydrates and remain high. You

Q Will I need to follow a "diabetic diet"?

A No—the basic principles of healthy eating for people with diabetes are the same as the recommendations for everyone else. You don't need to follow any restrictive meal plans or eat products labeled as "diabetic."

MAKING HEALTHY CHOICES
It's important to choose healthy, nutritious foods most of the time, but less healthy foods on occasion won't do you any harm—it is the overall balance of your eating that matters.

need to eat carbohydrate-containing foods because they are your body's main source of energy, but you can choose among the many types of carbohydrates and eat them in quantities that will balance with any pills and/or insulin you take. In this way, you will help your body deal with the carbohydrates.

■ **TYPE 1 DIABETES** If you have type 1 diabetes, matching your food intake to the action of your insulin is the way to maintain a healthy blood glucose level. For example, if you take a shorter-acting insulin, you will need to take it around the time that you are having your meals. You will also be taking a longer-acting insulin, and you may need to eat extra snacks to make sure that there is food available in your body when your insulin is working at its peak. The exact timing of your food and insulin together will depend on the type of insulin you take (see pp.82–101).

■ **TYPE 2 DIABETES** If you have type 2 diabetes, your body's ability to produce insulin effectively when you eat is impaired. Therefore, it is important to choose foods wisely so you have both fiber and good fats in the meal. Fiber and fats help slow down digestion, so that the demand for your body to produce insulin is gradual. Also, you should avoid eating large quantities of carbohydrate-containing foods all at once in order to reduce the pressure on your pancreas to produce large amounts of insulin.

If you are taking pills for your diabetes, you will need to take them as prescribed in relation to your meals. This is because some of these pills work by helping your body break down food more slowly, while other pills make your pancreas produce more insulin. Therefore, if you do not time your pills correctly relative to your meals, they will not be effective

Myth OR TRUTH?

MYTH
People with diabetes should never eat sugar.

TRUTH
It is unnecessary to avoid sugar altogether. You can take steps to limit your sugar intake by not adding sugar to food and drink and by avoiding sugary foods and drinks most of the time, but many foods (such as fruit) that contain natural sugars are excellent sources of beneficial vitamins and fiber.

"For years, the type of insulin I took dictated when I had to eat, because if I didn't eat I would wind up with low blood sugar. Now, with newer types of insulin and delivery mechanisms, I can match my insulin to when I want to eat." STUART

COMMENT If you find it hard to eat at the right times to match your insulin, you may be able to try one of the many new insulins available. The latest insulins cause fewer low blood sugar episodes and enable you to eat what, when, and how much you want. Ask your health professional for advice.

> If your routine is unpredictable or your usual eating pattern is disrupted, you may find that your blood glucose level is less well controlled.

and may cause hypoglycemia (see pp.102–109).

It is common to be overweight if you have type 2 diabetes. Therefore, you may also need to try to limit portions and choose foods that will help you lose weight (see pp.44–51). Having type 2 diabetes in particular is linked with an increased risk of developing hypertension (high blood pressure), high cholesterol, and circulatory disease. Eating a healthy diet can help reduce this risk.

Food, drink, and your day

An important part of your diabetes control is recognizing when you need to eat or drink in order to balance the effects of pills or insulin on your blood glucose level. If your routine is unpredictable, or your usual eating pattern is disrupted, you may find that your blood glucose level is less well controlled.

If you take insulin or pills to stimulate your insulin production (see pp.76–101), eating at regular intervals throughout the day is essential in order to avoid low blood sugar. If you inject insulin or take pills in order to increase the insulin in your bloodstream and you don't eat, your blood glucose level will fall. Some pills (see pp.76–81) and some forms of insulins (see pp.82–101) are now available that enable you to closely match your insulin to your food, making it less likely that you will have too much insulin in your bloodstream.

Eating meals containing carbohydrate at regular times throughout the day will "fuel" your body, help your digestive system function properly, and avoid sharp rises and falls in your blood glucose level. If you have only one large meal a day, your body will struggle to turn this into energy quickly enough to keep your blood glucose level balanced. A regular eating pattern is also more likely to

Q I am vegetarian and I'm also Muslim, so I sometimes fast for religious reasons. How do I cope with this and with my diabetes?

A The healthy eating principles remain the same whether you are vegetarian or are following any other special diet—for example if you eat kosher food, or if you have celiac disease or allergies to certain foods. If you find it difficult to find enough variety of foods to eat, you can seek professional dietary advice. When you fast, you may need to adjust the dosage of your pills or insulin for the period that you are fasting and the times that you eat. Ask your health professional for guidance. In general, fasting during pregnancy when you have diabetes is not recommended, because it can be harmful to you and your unborn child.

fit in with any pills or insulin that you take for your diabetes.

■ **TIMING YOUR FOOD WITH MEDICATION** Knowing when your pills or insulin will work and when your blood glucose level is likely to start falling is useful. For example, some pills may make your blood glucose level fall mid-morning or mid-afternoon. As a result, you might need to eat a snack at these times. If you cannot eat when you need to, perhaps because of long shifts or meetings at work, for instance, it may be necessary for you to use a different medication that will suit your routine better. Discuss this option with your health professional.

■ **SNACKING** Having diabetes does not automatically mean having to add snacks to your day—it may be that eating regular meals at certain times controls your blood glucose level well enough. Also, if you are trying to lose weight, you may not want to increase your calorie intake. However, if you are taking certain types of insulin or pills, you may need snacks between meals and before bed to keep your blood glucose level steady. Alternatively, you may simply want a snack because you are hungry. If this is the case, try to make sure snacks are not high in fat or sugar—a piece of fruit is much healthier than a cookie. Also, snacking should not mean you eat more food overall—by reducing what you eat at other times, such as by having smaller meals, snacks will not be extras but part of your normal daily food intake.

Food groups

Foods fall into three main groups: carbohydrates, proteins, and fats. Eating the right balance of foods from each of these groups on a daily basis will help keep you healthy. You also need to be aware of the fruit and vegetables, vitamins and minerals, fiber, and salt that you are eating. Finally, you need to know the sugar content of different drinks. Once you have a clear idea of which types of food are better for you and in what quantities, you will find that shopping, cooking, and choosing meals when you are eating at a restaurant will be far easier.

Carbohydrates

Carbohydrates are classified into two categories: "monosaccharides," which are also known as sugars, and "polysaccharides," also known as starches.

■ **MONOSACCHARIDES** These are sugars in their simplest form (also known as sucrose or glucose). Foods that are high in sugar include sweets, chocolate, sugary drinks, and some cakes. Because these sugars are usually in highly refined foods that contain white flour and saturated fat as well, they offer little nutrition. You should eat these foods only in small quantities and only occasionally. You do not need to avoid eating sugar altogether, because it is just another form of carbohydrate, and is present in many foods. However, careful checking of food labels and choosing foods that

MONOSACCHARIDES
Cakes and pastries contain monosaccharides. When you eat these foods your blood glucose will rise sharply.

have a lower sugar content will help you keep your blood glucose level better controlled.

■ **POLYSACCHARIDES** These foods include bread, potatoes, rice, pasta, cereals, and beans and legumes. Polysaccharides are also broken down into glucose, but the fiber that is present in whole grains and beans slows down digestion.

GLYCEMIC INDEX OF COMMON FOODS

Foods are given a GI number between 1 and 100, with glucose (sugar) scoring 100 because it causes blood glucose to rise very quickly—within 30 minutes of being eaten. You can use your blood glucose results to measure the GI rating of different foods. Individual brands can vary. The following are guidelines; note your own results.

LOW (below 55)	MEDIUM (55–70)	HIGH (over 70)
Apples	Melons	Dates
Bananas	Pineapples	Watermelons
Carrots	Beets	Rutabaga
Tomatoes	Sweet corn	Parsnips
Cereal with milk	Muesli	Cornflakes
Rolled oats	Instant cereal	Puffed rice cereal
Oat bran	Grape nuts	Wheat biscuit cereal
Cracked wheat bread	Whole-wheat bread	Brown bread
Mixed grain bread	Rye bread	White bread
Pita bread	Croissants	Bagels
Pasta	Brown rice	Instant rice
Instant noodles	Couscous	Mashed potatoes
Sweet potatoes	New potatoes	Baked potatoes
Potato chips	Muffins	Rice cakes
Peanuts	Digestive biscuits	Wafer biscuits
Popcorn	Muesli bars	Doughnuts
Orange juice	Cranberry juice	Glucose drink
Yogurt	High-fat ice-cream	Tapioca

Managing your carbohydrate intake

Knowing how much carbohydrate is contained in what you eat and how quickly certain foods will cause your blood glucose level to rise helps you choose the amount and types of food you eat. There are two common ways of managing your carbohydrate intake that work well together: the glycemic index and carbohydrate counting.

The glycemic index

The glycemic index (GI) is a ranking of carbohydrate-containing foods based on their effect on your blood glucose level. Foods that are digested slowly have a low GI rating, and foods that are quickly absorbed have a high rating. The index is useful because you can help keep your blood glucose level in the recommended range by monitoring the GI rating of your food. If you eat too many high GI foods, your blood glucose level rises sharply and falls quickly. For this reason, eating more low and medium GI foods than high GI foods helps to balance your blood glucose level.

However, the GI of a particular food only tells you how quickly or slowly it raises blood glucose when eaten on its own. You usually eat a mixture of foods at any one meal—bread is often eaten with butter or margarine, and potatoes with meat and vegetables, for example. Combining foods with different GI ratings changes the overall GI of a meal. Use the GI as a guide to help you choose low GI foods to include in a meal or snack to lower the overall effect on your blood glucose level and check the result with your blood glucose meter. If you eat a baked potato (high GI), for example, adding baked beans (low GI) reduces the overall GI of the meal, as well as helping to balance your meal.

The GI of a food is only one consideration. You need the nutrients in whole grains and fruits and vegetables to be healthy. If you are taking pills or insulin, eating only low GI foods might result in having more insulin in your system than you need. Some low-GI foods are also higher in fat—peanuts, for example—which might not be the best choice for large servings if you want to eat wisely.

Carbohydrate counting

Carbohydrate (CHO) counting is a way of tracking how much carbohydrate you are eating so that you can calculate how much insulin you need. You may have been taught carbohydrate counting as a method of blood glucose control. People taking pills may try to eat similar amounts of carbohydrate at set times each day, so their blood glucose level is about the same every day. With practice you can choose from all carbohydrate-containing foods, even when dining at restaurants.

Today, carbohydrate counting is used with newer rapid-acting insulins to give people more freedom in what they eat. If you take insulin you get to choose what to eat and then match your quick- or rapid-acting insulin

---

UNDERSTANDING CARBOHYDRATE CONTENT

The more carbohydrate you have, the more insulin you need to convert it into energy. Knowing how much is in different foods can help you decide how much of it to eat and adjust your medication.

AMOUNT	TYPE OF CARBOHYDRATE
10 g CHO	1 thin slice bread, 1 tablespoon uncooked rice, 1 plain cookie, 2 tablespoons baked beans, 1 small apple
15 g CHO	1 medium slice bread, 1 3 oz. boiled potato, 7–10 medium french fries, 1 medium pear, 1 medium grapefruit
20 g CHO	1 thick slice bread, 1 large croissant, 1 cup custard, 1 mango, 2 tablespoons raisins
30 g CHO	1 bagel, 1 cup bran cereal, 4 slices pineapple, 8–10 dried apricots

---

doses, via injection or insulin pump, to the amount of carbohydrate the food contains.

To establish your personal quick- or rapid-acting insulin to carbohydrate ratio, you need to find out how much insulin you need for every 10 g of carbohydrate (for example) you eat. If, for example, you need 1 mg of insulin for every 10 g of carbohydrate, your ratio will be

POLYSACCHARIDES
You should aim to include polysaccharides in every meal to give you the nutrients your body needs.

1 unit to 10 g carbohydrate. You can then use this to calculate how much insulin you need whenever you eat any carbohydrate-containing food.

If you are finding it difficult to control your blood glucose and you are prepared to carry out more frequent blood glucose testing and assess your food and insulin doses throughout each day, your health professional can help you find out more about using this method.

Proteins

Protein-rich foods include meat, fish, eggs, cheese, beans, and legumes. Your body needs protein to create, maintain and repair its cells but to eat a healthy diet, protein should make up only about a fifth of any meal. Protein has little effect on your blood glucose level, but when you are choosing which type of protein to eat, you can make healthier choices—for example, by ensuring that you do not eat red meat every day, or that you eat low-fat cheese, and include fish in your meal 2–3 times a week.

Fats

Fats are found in dairy products, such as milk, butter, and cheese, cooking oils, meats, and nuts, as well as in processed foods. Everyone needs to include some fat in their diet—it is an important component of many body cells and plays a key role in growth and development. However, it is recommended that women eat no more than 70 g of fat per day, and men no more than 95 g per day. The type of fat you eat is also important. You will find the healthiest fats in olive oil, canola oil, certain fish, seeds, such as flaxseeds, and nuts. A handful of almonds a day is as likely to help keep you healthy as the proverbial apple a day.

DIFFERENT TYPES OF FAT

Some types of fats are better for you than others, so it's useful to know which increase your chances of developing heart and circulatory problems and which (in small quantities) are beneficial to your health.

HEALTHIER FATS

MONOUNSATURATED FATS Found in olive oil and canola or rapeseed oil, and also in avocados, nuts, and seeds, these fats do not raise cholesterol levels (and are even thought to lower them). They are a healthier alternative to saturated fats (see below).

POLYUNSATURATED FATS The two groups of polyunsaturated fatty acids, omega-3 and omega-6. Omega-3 is found in oily fish such as salmon, flaxseeds, almonds, and walnuts. Omega-6 is found in sunflower, safflower, and corn oils. These fats are healthier than saturated fats, particularly omega-3.

LESS HEALTHY FATS

SATURATED FATS These are mainly found in animal products—cheese and the fat around a piece of steak are examples—but they are also found in coconut and palm oils. These fats raise blood cholesterol, which can lead to health problems including hypertension (high blood pressure) and heart disease.

TRANS FATTY ACIDS Often listed on food labels as "hydrogenated" or "partially hydrogenated," these synthetic saturated fatty acids are in many processed foods, such as cookies and cakes. They raise cholesterol levels, and eating foods that are high in trans fatty acids is linked to an increased risk of a heart attack.

Fats have little effect on blood glucose, but there are good reasons to limit your saturated fat intake when you have diabetes. Eating too much fat is linked to high levels of fat in the blood (hyperlipidemia), heart and circulatory disease, and stroke (see pp.206–211)—all complications of diabetes. Being overweight can also contribute to the risk of developing these complications, and fats are very high in calories. While dairy products can be high in fat, they also contain protein and carbohydrate and are a source of calcium and vitamins. To protect against heart and circulatory conditions, and also to help if you are trying to lose weight, choose lower-fat versions of fatty foods, such as fat-free or 1% (lowfat) instead of 2% or whole milk.

Vitamins and minerals

A healthy, balanced food intake provides all the vitamins and minerals you need. Whether you have diabetes or not, you do not need to take vitamin or mineral supplements unless your doctor or health professional advises it.

Fruit and vegetables

In addition to being low in calories and rich in fiber, fruit and vegetables are excellent sources of vitamins and minerals. For a healthy diet, your daily food intake should include at least five portions of fruit and vegetables—fresh, canned (in natural juice or water rather than syrup), frozen, or dried. A portion is one piece of fruit such as an apple or pear, a ½ cup of fruit juice, a ½ cup of vegetables, or 1 cup of salad. However, fruit and natural fruit juices also contain sugar (fructose), so more than one piece of fruit at a time, or more than a small glass of fruit juice a day, will raise your blood glucose level. Space out your fruit consumption throughout the day so that you gain the nutritional benefits without raising your blood glucose level too much.

Salt

Having diabetes increases your risk of developing hypertension (high blood pressure) and other circulatory conditions. Eating too much salt also increases this risk. If you have hypertension, too much salt can make it worse. Using less or no salt in cooking and not adding salt at the table will help you keep your salt intake within the recommended daily amount of no more than 2,400 mg of sodium.

FRESH FRUIT
Fruit is an ideal snack—it is relatively low in calories and full of beneficial vitamins—but if you eat too much at once, the fructose can raise your blood glucose level.

Practical tips

CUTTING DOWN ON FAT

- Replace butter or whole-fat margarines with lower-fat spreads, particularly products that contain monounsaturated fats.
- Avoid hydrogenated vegetable oils (trans fats).
- Use low-fat half and half, yogurt, or lowfat milk instead of whole-fat cream.
- Try to eat more fish and poultry than red meat.
- Choose lean cuts of meat and skinless poultry.
- Avoid fried foods.

Myth OR TRUTH?

MYTH
It's okay to eat a small banana, but a large banana will raise your blood glucose level.

TRUTH
The small banana contains carbohydrates, too. What matters is how much carbohydrate, protein, and fat is in a meal or snack. And everyone needs at least 5 servings of fruits and vegetables every day.

Fiber

There are two types of fiber, both of which are important to your health. Insoluble fiber, found in cereals and some vegetables, aids digestion and helps prevent constipation. Soluble fiber, found in legumes, oats, fruit, and some vegetables, slows down the digestion of carbohydrate. This stops your blood glucose level from rising too quickly after eating. It also helps reduce your cholesterol level. Aim to eat around 25 g of fiber a day.

Diabetic products and sweeteners

You may see foods labeled "diabetic" at supermarkets and health food stores. These products are not as beneficial as they sound because they usually contain the sweetener sorbitol, which is high in calories and makes your blood glucose level rise just as ordinary sugar does. In large quantities, sorbitol will also give you diarrhea. Diabetic foods are not recommended, since they do not help you control your diabetes.

Friends and relatives may buy you diabetic products because they don't know what you can eat, and they find the labeling reassuring. Let them know that it is fine for you to eat normal chocolate, sweets, cookies, and similar foods, as long as you don't eat them all the time or in large quantities. You can use artificial sweeteners instead of sugar to sweeten food and drinks, such as tea and coffee. These products

contain aspartame, saccharin, cyclamate, acesulfame K, or sucralose, none of which affects your blood glucose. However, these products are classed as food additives and have been tested for safety. Because of this, each type of sweetener has a recommended daily amount (shown on the label) that should not be exceeded.

Drinks

Sugary drinks such as sports drinks, cola, lemonade, and orange juice are digested very quickly, which is why it is recommended that you drink them when your blood glucose level is too low (see pp.106–108). For day-to-day drinks, choose sugar-free substitutes. Tea, coffee, and other hot drinks will not affect your diabetes, but drinking them with skim or lowfat milk will cut down on calories. Powdered drinks can have a high sugar content, so compare labels before you buy.

Q How much alcohol can I drink without affecting my health?

A The current guidelines state that, in general, men should drink no more than 2 drinks per day, and women, no more than 1 drink per day. One drink is equivalent to 1 single measure (35 mL) of whisky, a 125-mL glass of wine, or half a pint of ordinary beer. There may be times when you exceed the recommended amounts, however. As with many other things related to your health, an occasional lapse won't do any long-term damage.

ALCOHOL AND BLOOD GLUCOSE

Alcohol contains monosaccharides, so drinking will initially raise your blood glucose level—the higher the alcohol content, the greater the effect. In larger quantities, however, alcohol prevents your liver from releasing glucose from its stores, lowering blood glucose and increasing the risk of a hypo occurring.

DRINK	CALORIES	CARBOHYDRATE CONTENT	ALCOHOL CONTENT	EFFECT ON BLOOD GLUCOSE
Dark beer (1 pint)	140–185	9–14 g	4.5%	Dark beer causes an initial rise in your blood glucose level. Ordinary bitter has less effect on your blood glucose than strong or real ale.
Light beer, lager (1 pint)	170–230	7.5 g	3.2–4%	Lager causes an initial rise in your blood glucose level. Low-carbohydrate/diet lagers will not raise your blood glucose, but can be high in alcohol.
Glass (125 mL) dry white wine / sweet white wine	80–90 / 110–120	0.7 g / 7.5 g	9–14.5% / 9–14.5%	Dry and sweet wines contain similar amounts of alcohol, but dry wine has less effect on your blood glucose level because it contains less sugar.
Glass (125 mL) red wine	80–90	0.4 g	9–14.5%	Red wine contains less carbohydrate than white wine, but the effect on your blood glucose level is similar.
Single measure (35 mL) liquor	80	trace	40–75%	All liquors have similar amounts of alcohol and calories. On their own they do not greatly raise your blood glucose level.
Glass (35 mL) dry sherry / sweet sherry	58 / 68	trace / 3.5 g	15.5–20% / 15.5–20%	Dry sherries have less effect on your blood glucose than sweet varieties.

Using artificial sweeteners in drinks instead of sugar won't affect your blood glucose level.

■ ALCOHOL There's no reason why you shouldn't drink alcohol if you have diabetes, unless you have been advised not to because of other medical conditions or treatment.

However, drinking alcohol initially raises your blood glucose level because it contains monosaccharides. In larger amounts, it can inhibit your liver's response to hypoglycemia, which is to release glucose. This increases the risk of a hypoglycemic attack if you take insulin or insulin-stimulating pills or if you drink on an empty stomach. You can reduce the risk of having a low blood sugar level by having a meal containing carbohydrate before or while you are drinking alcohol. If you can't eat a meal, snack on sandwiches, chips, or cereal bars, particularly if you drink more than 2–3 units of alcohol. If you will be drinking a lot of alcohol and food might be in short supply, you may need a smaller dose of your pills or insulin on that day to reduce the risk of hypoglycemia. It is better to have a slightly higher blood glucose level for a short time than suffer a serious hypoglycemic episode that might necessitate hospital treatment.

Practical tips

INCREASING YOUR FIBER INTAKE

- Add extra fruit to breakfast cereals and yogurts.
- For snacks, have a piece of fruit instead of a cookie, and keep chopped raw vegetables, such as carrots, celery, and tomatoes, on hand in the refrigerator.
- Add beans (such as baked beans) to chopped meat and chili con carné (this will also reduce the meat and fat content of these dishes).
- Remember to count the carbohydrates.

QUICK AND EASY STIR-FRIES
Stir-frying is an excellent way of cooking vegetables and many other foods. Not only does it require very little oil, but the cooking time is very short, so food retains its nutritional content.

It is important to tell a friend what he or she should do if you have a low blood sugar level. People who don't know you might think you are drunk when you are in this state—they won't realize that you need help quickly if your blood glucose level falls too low.

Alcohol is high in calories, so you may need to cut down if you are trying to lose weight or avoid gaining weight. Mixers, such as tonic, cola, and lemonade, are high in sugar, so you should drink low-calorie alternatives to prevent your blood glucose level from becoming too high.

Healthier cooking

Having diabetes doesn't mean you have to forgo your favorite recipes. Instead you can adapt your cooking to reduce your overall fat and sugar consumption, include more fruit and vegetables, and generally make sure that your diet is healthy and well-balanced. There are low-fat, low-sugar substitutes for most ingredients in everyday dishes. There are also

healthier methods of cooking that will reduce calories without compromising flavor.

Recipe adjustment

Try the following ideas for cooking healthier meals:

- **SOUPS** Use more vegetables to increase fiber and reduce fat content. Avoid adding cream; use milk instead, since the extra fat is unnecessary.
- **PÂTÉ** Instead of cream and butter or margarine to bind pâté, use a combination of lowfat cream cheese and/or half-and-half.
- **CHEESE-BASED APPETIZERS** To reduce fat content, choose goat's cheese or feta cheese rather than cheese made from cow's milk.
- **SAVORY SNACKS** Lightly brush oil onto spring rolls, filo pastry snacks, or cheese in breadcrumbs and bake them in the oven instead of deep-frying them.
- **MINCE DISHES** Precook chopped beef or lamb and drain off some of the fat. If you are using strong flavorings (spices or curries), try using meat substitutes or soy products.
- **PIES** Pastry is high in fat, so use a very thin layer of pastry or make a mashed potato topping. Add herbs, chopped scallions, or chicken broth to a potato topping instead of butter.
- **CASSEROLES** Replace a proportion of the meat or chicken in a recipe with vegetables.
- **PASTA DISHES** Use tomato-based rather than cream-based sauces.
- **MAYONNAISE** Use a combination of natural yogurt and half-and-half or

milk instead of mayonnaise, which is high in fat.

■ **HOMEMADE ICE CREAM** Use heavy cream or milk instead of single or double cream.

■ **TRIFLE** Use plain sponge fingers; fresh, frozen, or canned fruit (in natural juice); low-fat cream cheese instead of cream; and a sprinkle of icing sugar if you need a sweetener. If you are using glazed fruit to decorate the trifle, rinse off the preserving sugar.

■ **TIRAMISU** Use virtually fat-free and reduced-fat cream cheeses in equal quantities instead of eggs and mascarpone cheese. You can still add a small amount of sugar.

■ **CHEESECAKE** Opt for low-fat soft cheese, add fresh fruit, and decorate with grated orange or lemon rind rather than cream.

■ **CRUMBLE** Use oats or whole-wheat flour for the crumble to increase the fiber content. Use more fruit filling and less crumble topping.

■ **SPONGE PUDDING** Use half the amount of sugar you normally use to make sponge.

■ **CUSTARD** Use fat-free milk, and add artificial sweeteners instead of sugar after cooking (not before, which will give the custard a bitter taste).

Cooking methods

Always try to grill, steam, or bake foods rather than fry or cook them in oils or fats. If a recipe requires frying, use cooking oil (see p.36 for healthier types) instead of butter. When cooking meat in the oven, place it on a rack to allow the fat to drain off. Adding herbs also helps bring out the flavor in food, thereby helping you reduce the amount of salt you add to your cooking. You don't have to miss out every high-fat or high-sugar ingredient from a recipe, however, especially if a small amount of that ingredient goes a long way. Parmesan cheese, for example, is high in fat but has a very strong flavor—you would need far more of most other types of cheese to achieve the same taste. Honey, too, may be high in sugar, but a small amount can sweeten a dish more effectively than a large amount of sugar. So if a recipe calls for small amounts of high-fat or high-sugar ingredients, go ahead and use it!

Eating out

There's no need to deny yourself the pleasure of eating out just because of your diabetes. Make healthy choices from the menu—keeping fat and sugar content to a minimum—when possible. If there is no healthy option, don't worry. You can adjust your

LOW-FAT CHEESECAKE
Reducing the fat content of a recipe doesn't make it any less tasty—but it does mean that you can continue to enjoy your favorite desserts as part of a healthy eating plan.

Taking a snack with you in case the service is slow will mean that you can avoid having a low blood glucose level while you are waiting.

medication to accommodate a rise in your blood glucose level if necessary. Even if you don't, the rise will be temporary and your blood glucose level will return to normal once you get back to your usual eating pattern.

The timing of a meal out may be different from your normal eating pattern, or you may not be able to predict exactly when you will be eating. You can get around this with some advance planning with regard to the timing of your pills or insulin injections.

You can alter the timing of your pills or insulin by about two hours without affecting your overall blood glucose level. If you delay your medication, however, your pills or insulin may continue working later than normal as a result. Make sure that your pills or insulin are always timed to coordinate with your intake

of food—for example, don't take insulin that will work in 15 minutes' time and then not eat for two hours. Wait until the food is served to take your insulin, or take a snack in case the service is slow. You can avoid having a low blood glucose level while you are waiting.

Choosing from the menu

If you eat out a lot, either socially or because of your work, you will need to pay more attention to the types of food you are eating. An endless round of fast food, pies, rich sauces, or three-course meals will cause your blood glucose level to rise and, in the long term, lead to increases in your weight, cholesterol level, and blood pressure. Although there are times when you don't have any choice, try to follow general healthy eating principles if you eat out regularly.

HEALTHY MENU OPTIONS

Every restaurant menu has options that fit well into a healthy diet. On the whole, vegetable-based dishes are healthier than meat dishes, but if you want to order meat, one of the "good" options will be lower in fat and calories. You also need to consider what foods accompany your dish, so that your meal is balanced. Ask for advice if you're unsure about ingredients, portion size, or cooking methods.

MEAT DISHES

GOOD: STEAK WITHOUT SAUCE

LESS GOOD: BEEF STROGANOFF

GOOD CHOICES: Steak without sauce; roast chicken (with skin removed); grilled lamb chops (with fat removed); stir-fried pork with vegetables.

LESS GOOD CHOICES: Beef stroganoff; beef pot pie; steak in gravy; fried lamb chops; burger with a bun.

FISH DISHES

GOOD: BAKED SALMON

LESS GOOD: FISH IN BATTER

GOOD CHOICES: Baked or poached salmon or tuna; grilled swordfish steak; smoked trout; tuna salad; paella with rice; fish stew such as bouillabaisse; seafood risotto.

LESS GOOD CHOICES: Fish in batter; deep-fried scampi; fish in cream sauce; fish in cheese-based sauce.

One way to eat out and stick to a healthy eating plan is to have only two courses for each meal. You can also ask for smaller portions and make sure that your meal contains a mixture of foods. Keep some of the following ideas in mind when choosing from the menu:

■ **APPETIZERS** Food that is deep-fried or drenched in sauce or oil is high in calories and fat. Choose a fruit- or vegetable-based appetizer instead.

■ **MAIN MEALS** If possible, ask for extra vegetables and a little less meat. Roast, sautéed, and mashed potatoes (which often include butter) are quite high in fat, so opt for baked potatoes instead. Order sauces in a sauce boat or side dish so that you can control what goes on your plate.

■ **DESSERTS** Fresh fruit is the healthiest option and is usually available even if it isn't on the menu. If you want to have your favorite dessert, however, ask for a small portion and some fresh fruit to go with it, or share it with a friend. Ask for any cream, custard, or sauce to be served separately.

■ **DRINKS** Low-calorie or diet drinks are far better for your blood glucose than high-sugar varieties. Fruit juices are also high in sugar.

CHANGING TASTES
Seeking healthier options on the menu can make you more adventurous about food and alter your tastes over time. You may come to prefer lighter dishes with less fat and healthier ingredients.

PASTA DISHES

GOOD: PASTA WITH VEGETABLE SAUCE
LESS GOOD: PASTA WITH CREAMY SAUCE

GOOD CHOICES: Pasta with pesto or tomato sauce; spaghetti Bolognese; pasta with tuna or smoked salmon or anchovies; seafood pasta.

LESS GOOD CHOICES: Pasta with creamy sauce, such as carbonara; beef lasagne, pasta with four-cheese sauce.

VEGETABLE-BASED DISHES

GOOD: VEGETABLE-STUFFED PEPPERS
LESS GOOD: VEGETABLE PIZZA

GOOD CHOICES: Vegetable-stuffed peppers; vegetable stir-fry; Spanish omelette; steamed vegetables with rice; ratatouille; grilled vegetable kebabs.

LESS GOOD CHOICES: Vegetable pizza; broccoli hollandaise; vegetable samosas; vegetable quiche.

Weight and diabetes

Maintaining a healthy weight is one of the most important steps you can take to manage your diabetes. Being overweight can raise your blood glucose level and cause hypertension (high blood pressure), increasing your risk of heart and circulatory problems. Where you carry excess weight on your body is also important. Find out whether you are a healthy weight for your height, why you may lose or gain weight when you have diabetes, and how to lose weight if you need to.

Myth or TRUTH?

MYTH
You can't lose weight if you have been heavy all your life.

TRUTH
It is possible for anyone to lose weight if he or she eats less and becomes more physically active. You need to take one step at a time, and set realistic targets to help you break any habits that you may have picked up over the years. If you find it extremely difficult to lose weight through healthy eating and physical activity, you may be given pills that will help you.

Why weight matters

Your weight can influence how easily you can manage your diabetes and can make a difference in the type and dose of any medication you take. Being overweight makes controlling your blood glucose level, blood pressure, and cholesterol more difficult and increases the risk of complications such as heart disease. Keeping your weight within the recommended range for your height (see p.46) or, if you need to, losing a little weight, has many health benefits.

Type 1 diabetes

Rapid weight loss is a common symptom of type 1 diabetes and a high blood glucose level (hyperglycemia). Once you begin insulin treatment, however, you should put the weight back on. If you have lost a lot of weight, you will probably need a low dose of insulin to begin with; once you start to regain weight, you may need to change the dose based on your own day-to-day blood glucose test results. Your weight will be checked at your annual examination and compared with the previous year to assess whether your insulin dose is too high—taking too much insulin can lead to weight gain (see pp.46–47).

Type 2 diabetes

You are more likely to develop type 2 diabetes if you are overweight because being overweight can make your cells resistant to the action of insulin. Four out of five people diagnosed with type 2 are overweight, so you may well have been advised to lose weight. Even losing a few kilos will make it easier to control your blood glucose level, lower your blood pressure and cholesterol, and prevent or delay the onset of future complications, such as heart disease.

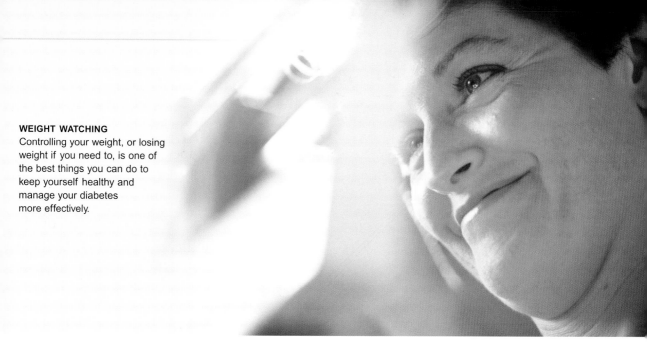

You are also likely to need a lower dose
of pills or less insulin, or you may be
able to control your diabetes without
any medication at all. If you are not
overweight, you may want to regain
some of the weight you lost or keep
your weight within a healthy range.

Why body shape matters

If you carry extra fat around your
abdomen rather than around your
hips, you have an increased risk of
developing heart and circulatory
problems. Even if you are overweight,
your risk of heart disease is reduced
if you have less fat around your
abdomen than around your hips. Use
the following calculations to assess
how your body fat is distributed:

■ **WAIST SIZE** Measure your waist
at the widest point. If your waist is
more than 102 cm (40 in) for a
man or 88 cm (34 in) for a woman,
you are carrying too much weight
around your middle.

■ **WAIST-TO-HIP RATIO** Measure your
waist and your hips at the widest
points and divide your waist size by
your hip size. For example, if your
waist measures 82 cm (33 in) and
your hips 103 cm (41 in), your
waist-to-hip ratio is 0.80. If the
result is more than 0.9 (for a man)
or more than 0.85 (for a woman)
you have a higher risk of developing
heart disease.

Is my weight OK?

To assess whether you are overweight
you need to measure your body mass
index (BMI), which is a ratio of your
weight to your height, expressed
in kilograms per meter squared. You
can either use a chart (see p.46)
or calculate your BMI yourself by
dividing your weight in kilograms by
the square of your height in meters.
For example, if you weigh 72 kg and
your height is 1.7 m, your BMI is
$(72 \div [1.7 \times 1.7]) = 25$.

> If you carry extra
> fat around your
> waist rather than
> around your hips,
> you have an
> increased risk
> of developing
> heart and
> circulatory
> problems.

WORKING OUT YOUR BODY MASS INDEX (BMI)

To find your BMI, measure your unclothed weight and your height. Trace a horizontal from your weight and a vertical line from your height on the chart below. The point at which the lines cross indicates the weight range you are in. You can then tell whether you need to gain weight, lose weight, or maintain your healthy weight.

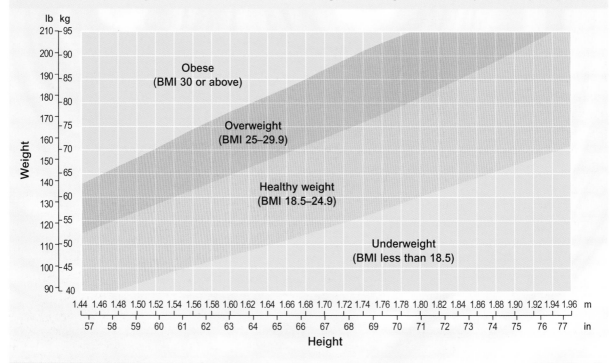

Weight

lb	kg
210	95
200	90
190	85
180	80
170	75
160	70
150	65
140	60
130	
120	55
110	50
100	45
90	40

Obese
(BMI 30 or above)

Overweight
(BMI 25–29.9)

Healthy weight
(BMI 18.5–24.9)

Underweight
(BMI less than 18.5)

1.44 1.46 1.48 1.50 1.52 1.54 1.56 1.58 1.60 1.62 1.64 1.66 1.68 1.70 1.72 1.74 1.76 1.78 1.80 1.82 1.84 1.86 1.88 1.90 1.92 1.94 1.96 m

57 58 59 60 61 62 63 64 65 66 67 68 69 70 71 72 73 74 75 76 77 in

Height

If you have a BMI of 25 or more, you are overweight; if you have a BMI of 30 or above, you are considered obese. Obesity carries an even greater risk to your health.

What causes weight loss?

Having diabetes can sometimes make you lose weight unhealthily. The most common reason for weight loss is a high blood glucose level, which means that your body is not using glucose properly for energy. Instead, your body begins to use fat from stores in your muscles and beneath the skin. If your diabetes continues to be uncontrolled, you will start to lose weight. Weight loss is more common and severe at diagnosis in type 1 diabetes, but it can also occur gradually in uncontrolled type 2 diabetes. You may also lose weight if you have other conditions possibly related to your diabetes that cause weight loss, such as an overactive thyroid.

What causes weight gain?

Some people with diabetes, and particularly those with type 2, put on weight. There are a number of reasons why you might gain weight:

• Taking more insulin than you need. This is because insulin causes your body to store glucose as glycogen in your liver and muscles and, if there is a plentiful supply, as fat beneath your skin. You may need to adjust your insulin dose to reverse this (see pp.90–95).

• Taking certain pills to lower your blood glucose level. Some types of pills can cause weight gain (see pp.76–81). You may need to consult your health professional.

• Consuming more calories than you need. You might be eating more because you are worried about having low glucose levels and want to prevent them, because you are having more snacks to balance with your pills, or perhaps because you have stopped smoking and are snacking to compensate. Or you may be eating comfort foods because you feel down or depressed. You may need to change your eating habits or eat a healthier diet (see pp.30–43).

• Being less active, perhaps because you are physically unable to exercise or because you find it difficult to fit physical activity into your day. You may need to plan how to increase the amount of activity in your day (see pp.52–59).

How to lose weight

If you need to lose weight, the best approach—and the way to keep the weight off—is to eat less and be more active. Bringing your weight into the recommended range for your height will be beneficial to your health: your blood glucose level and blood pressure will come down, your cholesterol level will improve, and you will look and feel better.

It is important to lose weight gradually: "quick-fix" diets that lead to rapid weight loss are unhealthy and you are less likely to keep the weight off. Your goal should be to lose about 0.5–1 kg (1–2 lb) per week. You may find that you lose more weight one week than you do the next. This is perfectly normal as your body adjusts to new habits.

You are much more likely to succeed in losing weight if you set practical, realistic goals for yourself. The first step toward successful weight loss is to look at what, when, and why you eat so that you can plan what to do differently.

Writing down what and when you eat and drink in a food diary can give you clues as to what unnecessary calories you are taking in and when. It will also show you whether your meals are spread evenly through the day and whether you are snacking unnecessarily between meals. When reviewing your food diary, ask yourself the following questions:

• Do I eat high-fat or high-sugar foods at certain times of the day?

AN ACTIVE LIFESTYLE
Control your weight by staying active and making sure that you don't consume more calories than your body needs.

MOTIVATING YOURSELF

- Empty your refrigerator and kitchen cabinets of tempting high-calorie foods and replace them with lower-calorie alternatives.

- Keep a record of your successes on a bulletin board. Don't focus only on your weight—include extra activity and how often you have resisted temptation.

- Put encouraging notes or inspirational pictures on your refrigerator and cabinet doors to remind you what you are aiming for.

- Ask for the support of a friend or family member you can talk to who will give you encouragement when you need it.

- Do I tend to taste food while I'm cooking?
- Do I use ordinary mixers with alcoholic drinks instead of low-calorie or diet versions?
- Do I dine out often, giving me less control over what I eat?
- Do I eat very large meals?

If you answered "yes" to any of the above questions, you could make changes right away to help you lose weight. To stay motivated on your weight-loss plan, set yourself small targets that you know you can achieve. Aiming to lose 1 kg (2 lb) by next week, for example, is far easier

to work toward than a goal of losing 18 kg (40 lb) by next year. Those 1-kg (2-lb) weeks will soon add up. Even if you only lose half a kilo (1 lb) in a week but are still following your food plan, your weight will continue to fall.

You may also find it useful to set goals related to your food intake rather than to your weight. For example, if you decide to cut out or cut down on certain foods during the week, you will feel more positive at the end of the week when you see that it has worked, particularly if your weight loss is a little slower than you would like.

USING A FOOD DIARY
Write down everything you eat and drink each day. After a week, review your diary in detail and plan what you could do differently. You could do this with the help of a health professional or friend. Don't forget to congratulate yourself for healthy eating, too!

August 1st

7:30am: bacon sandwich with 1 slice bacon, 2 slices white bread and lowfat margarine; tea with lowfat milk, banana

11am: small doughnut, can of diet soda

1pm: cheese sandwich with 2 slices bread; salad; apple; diet lemonade; 1 piece of chocolate; 1 bag cheese puffs

3pm: 1 piece of chocolate; grapes; coffee with lowfat milk

6pm: medium-sized turkey burger; 10 fries; tomato, cucumber, and lettuce salad; lowfat strawberry yogurt

10:30pm: cheese and crackers

Getting started

"The longest journey starts with a single step." Work through the following questions to help you come up with a plan that will work for you:

- How much weight would you like to lose?
- What specific changes are you going to make in what you eat?
- What specific changes are you going to make in your physical activity?
- How will you change your normal routine to include these changes?
- How will you find out how much weight you have lost each week?
- How will you motivate yourself to achieve your weekly goals?
- Who will you ask to help you stay motivated?
- What will you do at times when you aren't able to do what you have decided?
- When will you start your weight-loss plan?

Ask yourself whether what you have planned is realistic. If not, set yourself smaller goals that will bring you greater success. If you are successful once in doing what you have planned, you are likely to succeed again.

Once you feel confident that your weight loss plan is realistic for you, you might find it helpful to take time to list your strategies for overcoming temptation when your resistance is low. Keep the list handy so that you can refer to it whenever you need inspiration.

My experience

"I cut down my food and insulin, but ate complex carbs so I wasn't hungry. I had hypoglycemia at first and adjusted my insulin a lot, but in 8 months I lost 19 kg (42 lb) and needed less insulin overall." SHELLEY

COMMENT When losing weight, you may need to adjust your insulin dose often to avoid low blood glucose levels or having to eat more to balance your blood glucose. Once you've lost weight, you will need less insulin.

Calorie counting

The number of calories in food and beverages tells you their energy content. To maintain a healthy weight, you need to eat around 2,000 calories per day if you are a woman, and 2,500 calories per day if you are a man.

In order to lose approximately half a kilo (1 lb) per week simply by eating less, you will need to reduce the number of calories you consume by 500 a day. Fat contains double the calories that carbohydrate provides, so cutting back on fats in your diet is a good start. (See p.36 for the different types of fats and which ones

Q Does having diabetes mean that I shouldn't go on a low-carb, high-fat diet—even though it might help me lose weight very quickly?

A Diets that provide extremely different amounts of the main food groups may not be suitable for people with diabetes. A very low carbohydrate intake could cause you to become hypoglycemic if you take medication for your blood glucose level. If you think a specific eating plan is for you, you should discuss it with your health professional.

You may find it useful to set goals related to your food intake, rather than your weight.

you should choose.) However, even if you are eating less, you still need a variety of food types; excluding an entire type of food, such as protein or carbohydrate, is not healthy. Cutting out carbohydrate is particularly unhealthy since it is your main energy source, and your body will deplete its own energy stores in its attempt to compensate. Don't go below 1200 calories a day.

It is better to eat smaller portions of different types of foods instead of eliminating an entire food group. Make sure that you continue to include all the food groups in every meal and that you are getting all the nutrients you need. Eating fewer than three meals a day is not a good weight-loss strategy either—your body needs food at regular intervals to keep your diabetes under control. If you skip meals, you will not only compromise your blood glucose control, but you're also more likely to feel very hungry by the time you do eat, which can cause you to overindulge, or binge.

You may need to refer to a book that lists the calorie contents of foods. You may have to weigh some foods at first, to determine exactly how many calories you are taking in. You can then use your food diary to identify where extra calories are coming from and to decide how you can best reduce your calorie intake.

You can also look at the labels on packages and cans of food to find out the energy value. Knowing how to read a food label (see left) will help you make healthier choices overall—whether you are shopping for prepared meals or for ingredients in order to do your own cooking.

Some types of food and beverages are deceptively fattening, and you may be eating them without realizing how many hidden calories they contain. For example, fruit juice may appear to be healthy, but it is high in sugar; alcohol is high in calories; and most sauces are high in fat.

If you are physically active, you can allow yourself a few more

READING A FOOD LABEL
Compare labels on foods to make healthier choices and assess how much of which ingredients you are eating (ingredients are always listed in decreasing order of weight). If sugar, also called fructose or glucose, is an ingredient, look at its position on the list to gauge the quantity.
For more information visit www.healthyeatingisinstore.ca

Fat Compare different foods and choose those with a lower fat content (3g or less per 100g) to help you lose weight. Beware of saturated fats, too, which can raise your cholesterol level.

Sodium This is the salt content and although it won't affect your weight, limiting your intake reduces the risk of high blood pressure.

Carbohydrate The total amount of carbohydrate is given, and also how much of that is made up of sugars. A healthy amount of sugar per 100 g is 2 g or less—the higher the sugar content, the more chance of weight gain.

Fiber Choose foods with a higher fiber content—fiber not only aids digestion but helps you feel fuller.

Protein Protein is unlikely to cause large fluctuations in your blood glucose level, or affect your weight.

Calories This is useful if you are calorie counting to lose weight. Generally, opt for low-calorie products.

Serving size The serving size is important. Some cans or boxes may contain 2 or more servings, which doubles the amount of carbohydrate you're eating.

Nutrition Facts

Serving Size 1 cup (228 g)
Servings Per Container 2

Amount	%**Daily Value**
Calories 260	
Fat 13 g	20%
Saturated 4.5 g + Trans 0.5 g	25%
Cholesterol 30 mg	10%
Sodium 660 mg	28%
Carbohydrate 31 g	10%
Fibre 0 g	0%
Sugars 5 g	
Protein 5 g	

Vitamin A	4%	Vitamin C	2%
Calcium	15%	Iron	4%

calories and still lose weight. This is because physical activity burns calories while you are doing it as well as raising your metabolic rate (the rate at which your body uses up energy) over time. The number of calories burned depends on the intensity and duration of the activity. (For ideas on how to increase your activity level, see pp.52–59.)

Dieting and ketones

When you restrict your calorie intake, you force your body to burn its own fat stores for energy, which is why you lose weight. As part of this process, your body may produce toxic by-products known as ketones as it burns fat. These can make your breath smell fruity, rather like the smell of nail polish remover.

Producing ketones can be normal if you are losing weight, because it is an indication that you are burning fat. You may feel that producing ketones is a good sign because it means that you are succeeding at losing weight. However, for people with type 1 diabetes, producing ketones when you have a high blood glucose level is an indication of a dangerous lack of insulin (see p.113).

EATING BREAKFAST
Don't be tempted to skip breakfast as a way of saving calories—your body needs fuel to start the day. Have a smaller portion and include some fruit if you are trying to lose weight.

CUTTING DOWN ON CALORIES

You can make simple choices on an everyday basis that will cut out calories and help you lose weight without denying yourself the foods you like. Below are some low-calorie alternatives to high-calorie foods and drinks.

HIGHER-CALORIE FOODS	CALS	LOWER-CALORIE FOODS	CALS
100 g carbonara sauce	200	100 g tomato sauce	70
Small thick-crust pizza	350	Small thin-crust pizza	220
Bacon, lettuce, and tomato sandwich	502	Sliced turkey and tomato sandwich	274
1 can cream of tomato soup	216	1 can minestrone soup	93
Chicken breast with skin	300	Skinless chicken breast	190
50 g cheddar cheese	215	50 g cottage cheese	51
28 g blue cheese dressing	115	28 g lowfat Italian dressing	22
140 g cup yogurt	195	140 g lowfat yogurt	80
42 g salted peanuts	250	4 bread sticks	84
1 can soda	135	1 can diet soda	0
Small cappuccino	70	Regular-size espresso	4

Physical activity

Having a reasonably active lifestyle makes a huge difference to your general health and well-being as well as to your diabetes control. Whether you want to walk, dance, or run a marathon is up to you; if you are moderately active on a regular and long-term basis, you will feel the benefits. Find out how to get started if you haven't done much physical activity so far, how to devise a plan to meet your individual needs, and how to keep your blood glucose level balanced before, during, and after activity.

Practical tips

FITTING MORE ACTIVITY INTO YOUR DAY

• Walk or bicycle short distances instead of driving.
• Get off the bus one stop earlier and walk the rest of the way.
• Use the stairs instead of the elevator if you are only going up one or two floors.
• Walk up escalators.
• Incorporate a short walk into your daily routine, perhaps after lunch or in the evening.
• Do some extra gardening or housework.

Being more active

Being physically active is good for you, regardless of whether or not you have diabetes. It strengthens your heart, muscles, and bones, improves circulation, and helps control your weight. Being active also makes you feel fitter, healthier, and happier, partly because your body is working more efficiently and partly because activity raises levels of endorphins and serotonin, two brain chemicals that influence your mood and sense of well-being. If you are susceptible to depression (see pp.186–189), physical activity can help prevent or reduce its occurrence.

When you have diabetes, there are even more benefits to be gained from being active—150 minutes of moderate activity over at least three days a week can help regulate your blood glucose level and reduce the risk of long-term complications, such as heart and circulatory conditions.

If you have type 2 diabetes, regular activity helps reduce insulin resistance, which helps your own insulin work more efficiently. This may delay the need for increases in your pill dosage or the point at which you need to start taking insulin injections. If you have type 1 diabetes, being more active helps your injected insulin work more efficiently. As a result, you may be able to reduce your dosage.

How fit are you?

It is a good idea to assess your level of fitness before you start any regular activity. You may be surprised at the amount of activity you already do, or you may feel that you want to do more. Answer the following questions:
• Can you climb one or two flights of stairs without shortness of breath or heaviness or fatigue in your legs?
• Do you normally take the stairs rather than the escalator or elevator?

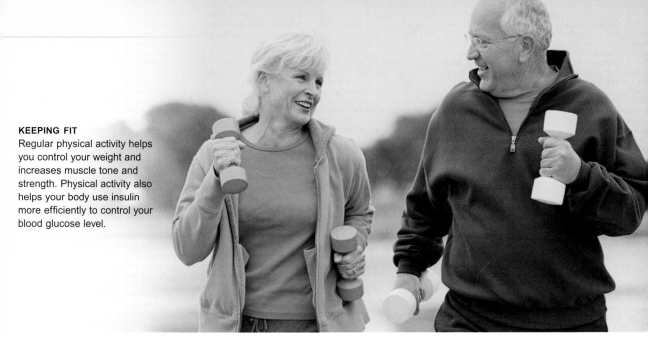

KEEPING FIT
Regular physical activity helps you control your weight and increases muscle tone and strength. Physical activity also helps your body use insulin more efficiently to control your blood glucose level.

- Would you walk 10 minutes rather than take the car?
- Are you able to converse comfortably during light to moderate activity, such as walking?
- Do you do 150 minutes of moderate physical activity that makes you sweat and breathe harder over at least three days a week?

If you answered "no" to any of the questions above, you could benefit from fitting more activity into your daily routine.

Getting started

Having diabetes places no restrictions on the type of physical activity you can do. If you haven't been active for some time, your best route is to start with any form of gentle activity, assess its effect on your blood glucose level and adjust your diabetes management accordingly. You can then build up your fitness gradually—once your body is used to regular activity, you

should aim to be active enough to feel warm and slightly out of breath. If you can sing while you are active, you could probably work harder; if you feel you are gasping for breath, slow down and catch your breath. You should not exercise so hard that you experience any pain.

Physical activity doesn't necessarily mean competitive sports or weight training. It also includes less vigorous pursuits such as walking, gardening,

---

CALORIES BURNED BY EVERYDAY ACTIVITIES

Day-to-day activities—indoor and outdoor—burn a surprising number of calories. Doing daily chores as part of your activity program is a good way of boosting your calorie expenditure.

ACTIVITY	CALS PER 30 MIN	ACTIVITY	CALS PER 30 MIN
Climbing stairs	330	Gardening, digging	240
House-cleaning	120	Mowing the lawn	140
Shopping	120	Cutting the hedge	120
Ironing	60	Gardening, weeding	105

MOTIVATING YOURSELF

- Set yourself realistic goals and gradually make them more challenging.
- Keep a record of your activity plan and your exercise program. It can show what you have already achieved and also help you identify where your plan worked and where it might need to be changed.
- Devise a reward system for yourself to celebrate your success at regular intervals.
- If a situation occurs to prevent you from being active, such as illness or a change in your working hours, a lapse doesn't mean that you have failed—simply revise your plan and get back to your activity as soon as you can.

or housework. Doing something energetic for 30 minutes a day, five times a week, improves your fitness and helps you control your blood glucose level more easily. You could spread your 30 minutes of activity throughout the day, or work out for an hour three times a week—whichever suits you best.

Building up your fitness

You may find it helpful to work out an activity plan, especially if you haven't been active for some time. The more detailed your plan, the more likely you are to succeed. You may be trying to make long-term changes in your approach to physical activity so it makes sense to look at the big picture right from the start.

Overall fitness is a combination of three factors: stamina, flexibility, and strength. If your aim is to improve your fitness, you need to do regular activity that makes your heart and lungs work harder (to build stamina), improves mobility in your joints (to increase flexibility) and develops your muscle strength.

If you want to lose weight, you may find that gentle activity, combined with changes in your food intake, is enough to achieve this. If not, however, you will need to burn more calories in order to lose weight. You could do this by increasing the intensity of the activity you do, by doing it more often or for longer periods, or by choosing an activity that by its nature burns more calories.

FITNESS BENEFITS OF DIFFERENT ACTIVITIES

When selecting a new activity, you can choose which aspect of your health and fitness to work upon: weight loss, stamina, flexibility, or strength. The fitness benefits of some suggested forms of activity are shown below. One square indicates a small benefit; four squares indicates an excellent benefit.

ACTIVITY	CALS PER 30 MIN	STAMINA	FLEXIBILITY	STRENGTH
Aerobics	215	■■■■	■■■	■■
Bicycling (fast)	280	■■■■	■■■	■■■
Golf	195	■	■■	■■
Hiking	200	■■■	■	■■
Jogging	245	■■■■	■■	■■
Swimming (fast)	300	■■■■	■■■■	■■■■
Tennis	210	■■	■■■	■■■
Walking (brisk)	180	■■■■	■■■	■■
Water aerobics	140	■	■■■■	■
Yoga	135	■	■■■■	■

Decide on your goal and then choose an activity that will help you achieve it. Consider the following to help you determine what you hope to achieve from being more active and how to go about it.

■ **WHY?** Decide what you want to achieve by becoming more active. Do you just want to feel healthier? Would you like to lose weight? Your goal will help you plan which type and how much activity you need to fit into your life.

■ **WHAT?** Think about the type of activity you want to do. If you enjoy it, you're more likely to find the time to do it.

■ **WHEN?** Be realistic about how often you will be able to do any form of physical activity. Will an activity be part of your normal day (for example walking to the store), or will you need to find extra time to do it? If you need to find more time, think about when it will be and how you can fit it around your other commitments.

■ **HOW?** Consider what might prevent you from carrying out your plan. For example, if the time that you set aside for your activity would usually be used to achieve other things, how will you still achieve those things?

■ **WITH WHOM?** Could you team up with a friend, partner, or family member? Sharing your exercise program with another person can often make the process of getting fit more enjoyable and give you the support and encouragement you need to stay active.

My experience

"Physical activity is difficult to fit into my day because I have a young child. But when I make time, I really notice the difference it has on my diabetes control for the next few days." SOPHIE

COMMENT   Most people with diabetes find that being active improves blood glucose control. If you are busy, you don't have to do formal exercise. Housework, gardening, and walking can help you stay active.

Warming up and cooling down

If your chosen activity is fairly intense, it is important to warm up before you begin. You can do this simply by doing your chosen activity at a slow pace for the first ten minutes. This prepares your muscles so that they work better and are less prone

SETTING THE PACE
Regular physical activity improves the flexibility of your joints and minimizes stiffness. To reap these benefits, you need to keep up your activity in the long term. You are more likely to continue if you enjoy whatever you do.

to injury. After your activity, you should cool down by decreasing the intensity of the exercise for the last ten minutes. Finish with gentle stretches—this is very important to prevent muscle pain and injury.

Managing physical activity and diabetes

When you have diabetes you need to be aware of the effect of physical activity on your blood glucose level and know what action to take to avoid the low and high blood glucose levels it can cause. The effect depends on how intense the exercise is (how many calories you burn, see box p.54) and how long you exercise. If you take insulin or pills to control your diabetes and you exercise intensively or for a long period, monitor your blood glucose level closely so that you can prevent your activity from causing a drop in blood sugar level.

Physical activity and blood glucose

When you exercise you need extra energy. Your body gets the energy it needs by converting the glycogen stored in your liver and muscles back to glucose. It also gets energy from the fat stored around your body.

Gentle activity for 10–30 minutes is unlikely to have much effect on your blood glucose level. However, with more strenuous activity, your blood glucose level will fall because of the extra glucose your muscles are using. When you stop the activity, your muscles and, to a lesser extent, your liver replace their glycogen stores by taking glucose from your bloodstream. The longer or more intense the activity, the more glucose is needed to replenish these stores, so your blood glucose level could be affected for several hours.

Managing blood glucose

Knowing when your blood glucose level is likely to fall will help you identify what, if any, action you need to take. If you are starting physical activity for the first time, test your blood glucose and check the effect of daily physical activities such as shopping and gardening. If you already do some regular activity, note

THE IMPACT OF ACTIVITY ON BLOOD GLUCOSE

If you are moderately active for 30 minutes or more, your blood glucose level changes throughout the activity. The more intense or long-lasting the activity, the greater the impact on blood glucose. Knowing about this helps you decide how to manage your diabetes.

DURATION OF ACTIVITY	EFFECT ON BLOOD GLUCOSE
0–10 minutes	Blood glucose level rises slightly as the body converts glycogen stored in the liver into glucose in the blood.
20–30 minutes	Blood glucose level falls slightly as muscles start to use up available glucose.
30–40 minutes	Blood glucose level could fall even further as more glucose is used up by the muscles to keep them working.
End of activity	Blood glucose level continues to fall as liver and muscles replace their glycogen stores by taking glucose from the bloodstream.

EATING TO CONTROL YOUR BLOOD GLUCOSE LEVEL BEFORE ACTIVITY

Here are some recommendations about whether you should eat—and, if so, examples of appropriate snacks—before you are physically active. Guidelines are based on the intensity and duration of the activity you do, together with your pre-activity blood glucose level in millimoles per liter.

TYPE AND DURATION OF ACTIVITY	BLOOD GLUCOSE BEFORE ACTIVITY	WHAT TO EAT 30 MINUTES BEFORE ACTIVITY
GENTLE: Walking or bicycling for less than 30 minutes.	5 or less	1 slice of bread or 1 piece of fruit.
	Any level above 5	Nothing.
MODERATE: Playing golf, leisurely bicycling, playing tennis, or swimming for 1 hour.	5 or less	1 slice of bread plus 1 piece of fruit.
	5.1–9	1 slice of bread plus 1 piece of fruit.
	9.1–15	Nothing.
	Above 15	Activity not advised until blood glucose level is lower.
INTENSE: Playing soccer or tennis for 2 hours. Vigorously bicycling or swimming for more than 1 hour.	5 or less	2 slices of bread plus 1 piece of fruit.
	5.1–9	1 slice of bread plus 1 piece of fruit.
	9.1–16	1 slice of bread or 1 piece of fruit.
	Above 16*	Activity not advised until blood glucose level is lower.

*If ketones are present, activity not advised if blood glucose above 14.

what effect that has and then compare the effect of more vigorous activity.

If you take pills or insulin, check your blood glucose level before and after your activity, and again a few hours later. If you are active for more than an hour, it is a good idea to check your blood glucose level in the middle of the activity. If you don't take pills or insulin, you won't need to make any changes whether your activity is intense or not, although

testing your blood glucose might be useful to see what a positive difference physical activity can make.

The following measures will help you keep your blood glucose controlled if necessary:

- If you have an elevated blood glucose level before you exercise, and it does not fall as you expect or rises even further, you probably don't have enough insulin to help your muscles use the extra glucose your body is producing. You may need to increase your pills or insulin dosage to make sure that your blood glucose is well controlled before you exercise.
- If you have type 1 diabetes and your blood glucose level is over 16 millimoles per liter (or 14 mmol/L if ketones are present), avoid exercise until your blood glucose is lower. When the level is this high, physical

Q Should I avoid physical activity because I have heart problems?

A Physical activity is particularly important if you already have heart problems, but do consult your health professional before embarking on a fitness routine. It is important that you start slowly and increase the amount of activity you do gradually over several weeks.

If you are active for more than an hour, it is a good idea to check your blood glucose level in the middle of your activity.

BEING PHYSICALLY ACTIVE SAFELY

- Keep sweets or soft drinks available in case your blood glucose level starts to fall while you are active.
- Record your blood glucose level, any changes you make to your pill or insulin doses, and any extra food you eat to help you plan for the next time you do similar activity.
- Take your blood glucose monitoring equipment with you if you plan to be active for an hour or more—you may need to do a test.
- Tell someone where you are going and what time you expect to be back if you are planning a long walk, run, or bikeride.

activity may cause it to rise even higher. To prevent a buildup of ketones, leading to ketoacidosis (see p.113), take your insulin and wait until it has had an effect.

- If you know that your activity will make your blood glucose level fall, you could reduce your dosage of pills or insulin beforehand.
- If your activity is unplanned, or if it won't make a big difference to your blood glucose level, you might have an extra snack beforehand rather than adjust your pills or insulin.
- If you have a low blood glucose level before your activity starts, you will need to eat something—ideally, half an hour before the activity.
- If your blood glucose level is still falling a few hours after activity, you will need to eat something then.
- If you are intensely active for more than an hour, you will need to refuel your glucose during the activity—energy drinks or sports bars will give your muscles the extra glucose they need. Energy drinks, every 1–1½ hours, will ensure that your body's glucose supplies do not fall too low.

Strenuous activity

If you are active for two hours or more, such as when participating in a marathon or competitive sport, you will need to pay even closer attention to your blood glucose level. If it is too high or low, your performance will be affected and you will get tired very quickly. Also, your blood glucose level might take up to

24 hours to return to normal, as your body replaces the glucose stores in your muscles. Regular testing is essential to monitor your blood glucose level and take action to reduce the chances of having a low blood glucose level.

There is no magic formula that will work for everyone, but the following recommendations help keep your blood glucose level steady during strenuous or long-lasting activity:

■ **MONITOR YOUR BLOOD GLUCOSE** If you are regularly active for more than an hour, test your blood glucose level before and after activity and also every 1–1½ hours during your activity. You may need to eat or drink something if your blood glucose level is falling. In competitive events, stress and excitement can make you produce hormones, such as cortisol and epinephrine (adrenaline). These hormones can also make your blood glucose level rise—another reason why monitoring is important.

■ **CARRY HIGH-SUGAR SNACKS** Having high-energy food or drink, such as sports bars, bananas, or non-diet

Q Does it make a difference where on my body I inject my insulin before physical activity?

A Yes. If you inject into the limb you will be using, the insulin will enter your circulation much more rapidly. This could cause your blood glucose level to fall too quickly. Choose a different injection site instead. For example, if you are planning to ride your bike, inject your insulin in your buttock or stomach rather than in your leg.

drinks, every 1–1½ hours, ensures that your body's glucose supplies do not fall too low. Drinking water will prevent dehydration.

■ **KEEP RECORDS** Knowing the effects of activity and food on your blood glucose level helps you to work out the best way to manage next time.

■ **LOWER YOUR PILL OR INSULIN DOSE** If you take pills that help your body produce more insulin (for example, sulfonylureas, see pp.79–80), you may need to reduce the dosage before your activity. Taking a lower dose of your longer-acting insulin the night or morning before the activity, or taking a smaller amount of your shorter-acting insulin with any pre-activity meals, or doing both, will reduce the chances of your having

a low glucose level during your strenous physical activity.

If you want to increase your muscle bulk or you are training for a specific event, such as a marathon, your program needs to be tailored to your needs. Endurance sports present specific challenges, especially for those with diabetes; you may need advice from your health professional.

Looking after your feet

Most physical activity involves putting extra pressure on your feet. Wear comfortable well-fitting shoes and check that they are appropriate for the type of activity you do. Always check your feet carefully for blisters and other damage before and after activity (see pp.128–130).

ENDURANCE SPORTS
Energy-consuming sports such as marathon running quickly use up glucose in your bloodstream, so you will need to keep refueling with glucose snacks or drinks as you go along.

Controlling your blood glucose

By keeping your blood glucose level within the recommended range you feel well and greatly reduce your risk of developing long-term complications.

This chapter gives you the information you need to work toward a blood glucose level that is as well controlled as possible. Frequent blood glucose monitoring and responding to test results accurately will help you manage your diabetes well.

If you take pills for diabetes, it is useful to know how these work and in what combinations they may be prescribed. If you take insulin to control your blood glucose, managing your regimen and learning to adjust your insulin doses when necessary puts you in control of your diabetes.

Even with close attention, instances of low blood glucose (hypoglycemia) and high blood glucose (hyperglycemia) are inevitable from time to time. By identifying the causes, however, you can help prevent them, and by recognizing the symptoms, you can treat them—either yourself or with help.

Monitoring blood glucose

Monitoring the amount of glucose in your blood is part of the daily care of your diabetes. It gives you information about how well you are controlling your blood glucose level, so that you can make adjustments to your treatment if necessary. To manage your blood glucose level in the most effective way, you need to know what level you are aiming for, what causes your glucose level to rise or fall, how to use your monitoring equipment properly, and how to interpret and act on the results.

Understanding blood glucose levels

The goal of treatment for all types of diabetes is to maintain a blood glucose level within a healthy range of 4–7 millimoles of glucose per liter of blood. Although you may experience symptoms if your blood glucose level is lower or higher than this, the only way to know for sure that your blood glucose level is within this healthy range is to take a sample of your blood and measure the amount of glucose in it. Regular tests will tell you how your blood glucose level is affected by the food you eat, physical activity, and the pills or insulin that you take for your diabetes.

If you start a new kind of diabetes treatment, monitoring your blood glucose gives you vital feedback about how well the treatment is working. Based on the results of your blood glucose tests, you will learn whether the type and dose of a new pill is correct or whether a new or revised regimen of insulin injections is working for you. Alternatively, if you have type 2 diabetes and you don't yet need pills or insulin, testing can help you learn about the impact of different foods, drinks, eating patterns, and activities on your blood glucose level.

An A1C test (see pp.66–67) is another way of monitoring your blood glucose level. This test is generally performed at your annual

BLOOD GLUCOSE TESTING
Some blood testing strips are designed to be read visually, but most are designed to be inserted in a blood glucose meter, which gives a more precise and accurate reading.

checkup (see p.26) and once or twice more over the course of the year—and may be done more frequently if your treatment changes.

Monitoring blood glucose

There are two ways of day-to-day blood glucose monitoring: testing your urine for glucose or testing your blood. In the past, urine testing was the standard way to monitor diabetes. A urine test result of negative or 0 percent glucose is the goal, but your kidneys filter glucose into urine only when your blood glucose level is around 10 millimoles per liter or higher, so a positive urine test only tells you that your blood glucose level is very high. A urine test doesn't tell you when:

• Your blood glucose level is slightly elevated (7–10 millimoles per liter).
• Your blood glucose level is low. Consequently, you can't exert very tight control over your blood

glucose level and you don't get the information you may need to avoid hypoglycemia (see pp.102–109). Consult your health professional to learn how to monitor your blood glucose using a blood glucose meter. There are many types of these meters, all with different options, so you need to pick a meter that fits your lifestyle and blood glucose goals. The only time that you use urine testing is to check for ketones. Check for ketones whenever you are sick or your blood glucose is running high. The procedure for testing your blood gives more precise results and is much more commonly used. This procedure is described on pp.70–73.

How often should I check my blood glucose level?

The general recommendations for useful times to test your blood glucose level are as follows:

If you start a new kind of diabetes treatment, monitoring your blood glucose gives you vital feedback about how well the treatment is working.

- Before each meal, to find out your blood glucose level when it is least affected by food.
- Two hours after each meal, to find out how well your body has used the glucose from your meal.
- Before you go to bed, in order to find out whether you need to take any action to keep your blood glucose well controlled during the night.

These seven options allow you to build up information about what happens to your blood glucose level at different times of the day (and in response to food). This will help you identify your usual blood glucose level at these times and will give you the opportunity to take action if your blood glucose level is either too high or too low. On some days, you may test at all these times or even more; on other days you may do just a few tests or even none at all. The factors that influence how

many tests you decide to do each day are as follows:

■ **TYPE OF TREATMENT** You may choose to test at times when your medication (insulin or pills) is working at its maximum or minimum effect, to make sure that your blood glucose level is not too high or too low at these times. If you do not take any glucose-lowering medication, you may test at times that measure the effects of different foods, timings, and physical activity.

■ **THE INFORMATION YOU REQUIRE** Sometimes you may choose to test more frequently than usual because you want to find out how your blood glucose responds to a specific situation, such as going for a mile-long walk, eating a particular type of food, or taking a new type of diabetes pill.

■ **GUIDANCE FROM YOUR HEALTH PROFESSIONAL** You may be given specific information by your health professional about how often to test your blood glucose level. This is based on an assessment of how well your diabetes is controlled. Sometimes you might be asked to test more frequently—for example, before an appointment with your health professional so that you can both make an accurate appraisal of your blood glucose control.

PLANNING A ROUTINE
The number of tests you do each day is up to you, but testing regularly and at standard times can give you a much clearer understanding of what affects your blood glucose level and can enable you to identify patterns.

Test before breakfast | Test 2 hours after breakfast | Test before lunch | Test 2 hours after lunch | Test before dinner | Test 2 hours after dinner | Test before bed

| 07:00AM | 08:00 | 09:00 | 10:00 | 11:00 | 12:00 | 1:00PM | 2:00 | 3:00 | 4:00 | 5:00 | 6:00 | 7:00 | 8:00 | 9:00 | 10:00 | 11:00 |

Breakfast | Lunch | Dinner | Bedtime

■ **LEVEL OF CONTROL** If it is very important that you achieve a blood glucose level of less than 7 millimoles per liter at all times, you need to test frequently so that you can act on the results. This level of control is necessary in certain situations, such as when you are planning a pregnancy, or if you have early signs of long-term complications.

Blood glucose levels to aim for

Blood glucose is measured in millimoles per liter of blood and, whatever type of diabetes you have, the recommended blood glucose level to aim for is 4–7 millimoles per liter. This is close to the blood glucose range of a person without diabetes. A blood glucose level within this range keeps you feeling well and helps protect you from long-term complications. There are occasional exceptions to this recommendation; your health professional can guide you on these. For example, if you have difficulty recognizing hypoglycemia (see p.106), you may be advised to keep your blood glucose level up to or even higher than 10 millimoles per liter for a period of time.

When monitoring is especially important

Monitoring your blood glucose is always important, but there are times when you may need to be more vigilant than usual.

■ **PHYSICAL ACTIVITY** If you are increasing your physical activity or

FACTORS THAT AFFECT BLOOD GLUCOSE

These everyday factors have an influence on your blood glucose level. If you understand their effect, you can take action to prevent your blood glucose level from rising too high or falling too low.

FACTOR	EFFECT
Carbohydrate foods; sugary soft drinks	Raise blood glucose. How quickly and how much depends on the type and quantity.
Physical activity	Lowers blood glucose by helping insulin to work more efficiently and using up energy.
Insulin injections	Lower blood glucose. How quickly and for how long depends on the type of insulin.
Diabetes pills	Lower blood glucose.
Stress	May raise or lower blood glucose, depending on the circumstances.
Illness	Raises blood glucose.

doing vigorous exercise, testing before, during, and in the few hours after (blood glucose can continue to fall hours after exercise), enables you to act quickly if your blood glucose level falls too low.

■ **CONCEPTION AND PREGNANCY** A high blood glucose level in the few months before conception or during pregnancy can have an adverse effect on your baby's development. Tight blood glucose control, avoiding even occasional high levels above 7 millimoles per liter, is critical.

■ **LONG-TERM COMPLICATIONS** If you develop the early signs of any long-term complications of diabetes, tight control of your blood glucose level can prevent problems from developing further and may help improve them.

■ **AN UNPREDICTABLE LIFESTYLE** If you have a social life or job in which your

Myth OR TRUTH?

MYTH

If I test my blood glucose first thing every morning, that tells me how well controlled my diabetes is.

TRUTH

If you do one test a day, you need to vary the times you do it in order to obtain information about your blood glucose level at different times of the day.

ON VACATION

A different routine, climate, and activity level, as well as new foods and eating habits, all affect your blood glucose level.

routine changes a lot, or if you do shift work, frequent testing tells you what effect this has on your blood glucose level and allows you to adapt the way in which you look after your diabetes accordingly. Even if your routine changes only for a day or two, it's important to be aware of the effect of this has on your blood glucose level.

■ **DRINKING ALCOHOL** Alcohol can cause your blood glucose level to rise initially, then fall; the more alcohol you drink, the greater the fall. Testing while you are drinking and a few hours afterward can warn you of possible hypoglycemia.

■ **ILLNESS** Illness can cause your blood glucose level to rise very high. Frequent testing, at least every four hours, may be necessary in order to give you the information you need to correct your blood glucose level and prevent you from feeling even worse.

■ **VACATIONS** Your routine may change when you are on vacation. Your food and alcohol intake and your levels of activity and stress are all likely to vary from the usual levels. Frequent testing will tell you the impact of these factors on your blood glucose level so that you can respond.

■ **FREQUENT INSULIN ADJUSTMENT** If you have type 1 diabetes and you fine-tune your insulin doses to your body's requirements, either by injection or using a pump, you need frequent information about your blood glucose level. This enables you to choose an appropriate dose of insulin based on what you are going to eat, or have just eaten, or your blood glucose level at the time. If you manage your diabetes in this way, you may need to test immediately before and two hours after every meal.

The A1C test

Apart from testing yourself, there is another important way to gather information about your blood glucose level: the A1C test (each letter is pronounced separately). This is a laboratory test performed by your health professional at regular visits. The Canadian Diabetes Association recommends a visit to the doctor approximately every 3 months to get an A1C blood test. The test involves analyzing a blood sample from your arm. The A1C test is not affected by anything that you have recently eaten or drunk. It measures the amount of glucose attached to the hemoglobin in your blood and gives an average

Q I've heard that you can buy home A1C testing kits. Is this a more advanced version of my existing blood glucose meter?

A No. An A1C test is different from your everyday blood glucose tests —it measures your control over a 6–8-week period rather than measuring your blood glucose at the time of testing. Whereas blood glucose levels can vary considerably at different times of the day, A1C values do not fluctuate so widely. Make sure your doctor discusses your A1C values with you, to determine whether you are in the normal range.

picture of your blood glucose level over the previous 6–8 weeks.

If you have an A1C test result of 7 percent or lower, this indicates good blood glucose control and is related to a reduced risk of developing long-term complications. A higher result than this, however, may indicate that your blood glucose level needs to be more tightly controlled—discuss this with your health professional to work out what changes you could make.

Monitoring equipment

Specialized equipment is available for testing your blood glucose level. The most common method of testing is to insert a blood testing strip into a blood glucose meter, then obtain a blood sample using a lancing device, and apply the sample to the testing strip to obtain a reading. Your health professional can help you decide what type of equipment is best for

you, or you may obtain information from books, the Internet, or the Canadian Diabetes Association (see p.218). When you decide on the right meter, make sure you receive the proper training from your diabetes health care team. Meters can be purchased at most pharmacies.

Lancing devices

Most lancing devices consist of a hand-held tube, containing a spring, into which you put a needle known as a lancet. A dial on the lancing device enables you to choose the depth to which the needle penetrates (a child would need a shallow setting, such as 1, whereas an adult with thick skin would need a deeper setting, such as 4). After setting the depth, you hold the device against the side of your fingertip and press a button to release the lancet, which pricks your skin. Some lancing devices are designed to

LANCING DEVICES
A wide range of lancing devices are available, all of which enable you to obtain a blood sample discreetly and with minimum discomfort. You load a lancet into the device, select a depth setting, prime the lancet for action, and press the release button to prick your finger.

Priming tube or handle

Button to eject lancet after use

Priming button

Depth selection indicator wheel

Spring release

Spring release

Depth selection dial

Depth selection dial

Release button

Lancet and spring cover

Lancet and spring cover (twists to prime)

Lancet and spring cover

Standard lancing devices

Priming tube or handle | Lancet holder | Lancet | Disposable cap | Lancet and spring cover with depth setting

LOADING A LANCET INTO A DEVICE

To insert a lancet into a lancing device, detach the end cover of the device, insert the lancet into the lancet holder, twist off the lancet's protective cap, and screw the device together again. The priming handle pulls the lancet back, ready to be released.

Lancets are designed to be used only once to avoid infection and also to make sure the needle is as sharp as possible.

take blood samples from areas of your body other than your fingertip, such as your forearm. Lancing devices come in a pack with a blood glucose meter and can also be bought separately. There are devices that use a laser to obtain a blood sample through your skin, but they are currently more expensive than other lancing devices, and are not yet in common use.

Lancets

Small, fine needles, known as lancets, are used with a lancing device to prick your skin and draw a small amount of blood. You insert the lancet into a lancing device, usually by unscrewing part of the device and screwing it together again. Lancets are designed to be used only once to avoid infection and also to make sure the needle is as sharp as possible—the sharper the needle, the less pain it causes. Some lancets are universal, which means they fit most lancing devices. Others are specifically made for one type of device. Make sure that the lancets you have are compatible with your lancing device.

Blood testing strips

Once you have obtained a sample of blood you put it on a blood testing strip. A pack of blood

testing strips usually contains 25 or 50. Always check the expiration date of the blood testing strips before use —out-of-date strips do not give an accurate result. Individually packed strips usually last about 2 years. Loose strips in a pot usually last a month after opening (it's useful to make a note of the date when you open a new pot of strips). Most blood testing strips are designed to be inserted into a blood glucose meter, but some are designed to be read visually (see p.73).

Blood glucose meters

Battery-operated devices known as blood glucose meters analyze the amount of glucose in the blood sample on your testing strip and then display

Testing strip

Strip holder

Memory button

Code button

Settings button

Memory button

Strip holder

Testing strip

Standard meter

Standard meter

the result in millimoles per liter on a small screen. There are two main types of meters. With one type, you insert one end of a testing strip into the meter then apply your blood to the other end. The end of the strip inside the meter contains an electrode, which is read electronically by the meter. With the other type of meter, you insert the end of the strip into the meter, then apply blood to the pad of the strip. The meter performs an electronic analysis of the changing color of the pad.

Both types of meters are highly accurate (provided you follow the manufacturer's instructions) and give results ranging from 0.6–33.3 millimoles per liter.

When choosing a meter, it is worth considering the following features.

Q **If my blood glucose meter gives me a result in the display screen, can I assume that this is always correct?**

A To get an accurate result, you must use the meter in the way that the manufacturer recommends. If you haven't calibrated your meter properly, or you use out-of-date blood testing strips, the meter will not give you an accurate result. Your meter may also give you an inaccurate result if your blood sample is too small or if it is contaminated— for example, if the site from which you obtain your sample is not clean.

■ **SIZE** Some meters are smaller and more compact than others. If you have arthritis or any other condition that affects your dexterity, you may find a larger meter helpful.

■ **RESULT DISPLAY** Meters with large displays may be easier to read if you have poor eyesight. Some meters

BLOOD GLUCOSE METERS
Blood glucose meters are available in various shapes and sizes to suit individual requirements. Some provide standard functions; others offer additional features or incorporate another device.

Testing strip

Strip holder

Settings button

Memory button

Memory button

On/off and memory button

Backlight

Code button

Memory button

On/off button

On/off button

Lancet

Insulin cartridge holder

Testing strip

Testing strip

Testing strip

Meter with insulin delivery device

Meter with built-in blood testing strips

Meter with lancing device

give just the test result, others give you the date and time.

■ **MEMORY** Meters vary greatly in the number of results they can store. Some can store 10; others can store up to 450. A large memory is useful if you're often in situations that make it difficult to write down your results.

■ **COMPUTER DOWNLOAD FACILITY** Some meters have a facility that allows you to download your results and analyze them on a computer. This enables you to view your results over a period of time in graph or table form.

■ **AVERAGES** Many meters provide you with an average of your readings, for example over the previous 7, 14, or 28 days.

■ **SIZE OF BLOOD SAMPLE** The amount of blood you need to put on your strip can vary from 0.3 to 10 microliters. If you find it difficult to obtain blood, it may help to choose a meter that needs a smaller sample.

Q Is there a device that can continuously monitor my blood glucose level?

A There are two devices available for continuous testing: a watch-like device that you wear on your wrist and a machine that is connected to a needle in your abdomen. Neither are widely used because the technology is still being developed and you therefore still need to do conventional blood glucose tests in conjunction with continuous testing. Also, the device that uses a needle in your abdomen doesn't produce on-the-spot readings—you need to download information to a computer before you can access your results.

■ **TIMING** After you have applied blood, meters can take 5–45 seconds to give you a result. A meter with a shorter analysis time may make it easier for you to test when you are busy.

■ **TESTING SITES** All meters can analyze blood from your fingertips but some can also analyze blood from your forearm, the palm of your hand, or your abdomen. If you find that your fingers get sore from testing or you use your fingers in your work and taking blood from them is difficult, a choice of testing site can be useful.

■ **ADVANCED FEATURES** Some devices combine a blood glucose meter with an insulin delivery device. Others measure both blood glucose and blood ketones (see p.113), or combine a blood glucose meter with a lancing device. Ask your health professional for more information about different devices in order to help you decide whether another device would be better for your purposes.

Performing a blood glucose test

There are two methods of performing a blood glucose test: you can use a blood glucose meter to obtain a precise reading; or you can do a visual test, which gives you results as a range. It is much more common to use a meter than to do visual testing, so your health professional will probably recommend that you use a blood glucose meter. Whichever method you use, by following the manufacturer's instructions that come with your equipment, you will ensure your results are accurate.

Using a blood glucose meter

Depending on the type of meter you have, the procedure for carrying out a blood test will vary, which is why it's very important to follow the instructions that come with your machine. However, with most machines, you will need to do the following to obtain an accurate result.

- If you are starting a new pot of blood testing strips, prepare your meter by calibrating it. You may need to carry out a quality control test if you are using the meter for the first time or you haven't done a control test for over a month (see box, below).
- Insert a blood testing strip into your meter—unless the meter contains strips, or you need to apply blood before inserting the strip (your instructions will tell you which method to use).
- Obtain a blood sample (see p.72).
- Apply blood to the testing strip and wait for the meter to display your blood glucose level.

If you insert your strip and then take too long to apply your blood,

PREPARING A BLOOD GLUCOSE METER FOR USE

Because blood testing strips vary from batch to batch (they may contain different amounts of chemicals), you need to calibrate most meters every time you start a new pot of strips, to guarantee an accurate result. You should also test your meter at least once a month with a quality control solution. The solution contains a known amount of glucose, enabling you to check that your meter is measuring blood glucose correctly.

1 If your meter has a coding chip provided with the strips, insert it into the slot on the meter. If it has a coding strip, insert this into the meter, then remove it once the code has been registered. If it has a code (C) button, insert the strip, then press the button until the code matches the new pot of strips.

2 When you insert a test strip, compare the code number on the display with the number printed on the test strip pot. The two numbers must be identical. If they are not identical, you need to repeat the procedure until the correct code number is displayed.

3 To test using the quality control solution, apply the solution to the test strip in the same way as you would apply your blood, then compare the control solution result with the range printed on the test strip or control solution package. The result should fall within this range.

OBTAINING A BLOOD SAMPLE

The blood test forms part of your day-to-day routine when you have diabetes. Although your finger is the most common site for extracting blood, you can also test blood from your forearm, the palm of your hand, or your abdomen—if your equipment is designed to test blood from these sites. Following these steps will help ensure that you get an accurate reading from your blood glucose test.

1 Wash your hands and then rub or shake them to maximize your circulation. Put a fresh lancet into your lancing device and carefully remove its disposable cap.

2 Replace the device's cover and turn the dial to set your preferred depth level. Low numbers indicate a shallow depth, higher numbers mean that the lancet goes deeper into the skin.

3 Take a fresh blood testing strip out of its package or pot. Switch on your blood glucose meter if you use one, or insert the test strip into the meter to switch it on, according to the manufacturer's instructions.

4 Put your lancing device firmly against the side of your finger. Press the button on the side or the end of the device to fire the lancet. Move the lancing device away from your finger and wait a few seconds for the blood to flow.

5 If a drop of blood doesn't appear, apply pressure to the base of your finger near the knuckle, moving downward, to assist blood flow. If you still can't get enough blood, start again using another finger and a new test strip, and increase the depth setting if necessary.

6 When you have enough blood, apply it to the pad on the end of the testing strip. Depending on the type of strip, wait 5–45 seconds for your meter to display your blood glucose level.

your meter will switch itself off in order to save battery power. However, once the testing strip has blood on it and is in the meter, a built-in timing device takes over.

Visual blood glucose testing

If your meter malfunctions or is damaged, estimates of blood glucose can be obtained by visually reading the strip, although this is only recommended in emergency situations:

- Put a single drop of blood on a pad at one end of the strip (you need specially designed strips for visual testing). Make sure that the pad is covered with blood and note the exact time—you will need a watch or clock with a second hand or a digital display showing seconds.
- Leave the blood on the pad for the time specified in the manufacturer's instructions (usually 1–2 minutes), then blot or wipe it off using a tissue or cotton as recommended.
- After a second period of time has elapsed (refer to the instructions), read the result by comparing the color of the pad with the color chart on the pot.

The timing of all stages of visual blood glucose testing is critical. For example, if you wait longer than the specified time to compare the test strip against the color chart, the test strip may continue to change color and give you an inaccurate result.

Unlike a blood glucose meter, which presents your blood glucose level as a precise figure, the results

My experience

"I aim for levels of 6–7 millimoles per liter since I am trying to get very tight control. I feel hypoglycemic if my levels are 4 or below, and thirsty if my levels are 9 and above." SHELLEY

COMMENT Keeping good control of your diabetes helps you to avoid symptoms on a day-to-day basis. But even if you don't have symptoms, good control is important to prevent health problems in the future.

using visual testing are given as a range. For example, your blood glucose level might be in the range of 2–4, 4–7, 7–9, 9–11, or 11–17 millimoles per liter. This can make it difficult to know exactly how and to what extent to adjust your treatment. Another drawback of reading the results from a color chart is that it is difficult if you have poor eyesight.

Talk to your health professional about learning how to use a blood glucose meter.

Keeping a monitoring diary

It is important to record the results of your blood glucose tests so that you can see whether your blood glucose level fluctuates over the course of a day or a week.

A monitoring diary is designed for this purpose. It provides space for you to enter the results of seven or more blood glucose tests a day, together with the date and time and any relevant notes, such as what activity you were doing if you were feeling hypoglycemic. You can also note the time and dose of your pills or insulin (see p.91).

Practical tips

ENSURING ACCURATE TEST RESULTS FROM YOUR METER

- Read and follow the manufacturer's instructions about the features and use of your meter.
- Wash and dry the site you intend to take blood from. Dirt or food traces on your skin can produce an incorrect result.
- Make sure that you calibrate your meter each time you start a new pot of testing strips.
- Always use a new testing strip for each test.
- Don't "top up" blood on your strip if your equipment isn't designed for this. Use another strip and try again.

My experience

"Five tests a day means sore fingers! But it helps me stay in control of my disease and have the degree of flexibility that I want in my life." SOPHIE

COMMENT Monitoring is the only way of knowing what your blood glucose level is so that you can take action to keep it controlled. It can mean sore fingers, but it is now possible to obtain blood from other sites, too.

Responding to test results

If you keep your monitoring diary up-to-date, you can examine your blood glucose readings over a period of days or weeks and decide what, if any, action you need to take in response. Rather than focusing on the occasional high or low result, look for patterns. If you have a meter that you can use in conjunction with a computer, you can look at your results in graph or table form. Is your blood glucose level always high or low at a particular time of day? The ideal range for your blood glucose level is 4–7 millimoles per liter. If it becomes clear from your monitoring diary that your results are rarely or never in this range, or are constantly swinging between high and low, you can take corrective action by paying more attention to the type or amount of food you eat (see pp.30–43), being more active (see pp.52–59), or changing the dose of your pills (see pp.76–81) or insulin (see pp.90–95). If these measures don't work or you don't know why your blood glucose level is erratic, contact your health professional even if you are not due for an annual or routine review. You may need a change to your pills or insulin regimen.

USING A MONITORING DIARY
Recording your test results helps you spot patterns and shows you how different foods, activity levels, and adjustments to your pills or insulin, if you take them, affect your blood glucose level.

High blood glucose readings

A single high reading that is above 7 millimoles per liter with no obvious cause, whatever the level, will happen from time to time and you do not need to take any action. Repeated high readings over a day or more need to be dealt with, however.

The first step is to identify the cause (see box, right) and then act accordingly. So, for example, if your blood glucose level is higher than usual because a muscle strain injury has prevented you from being as

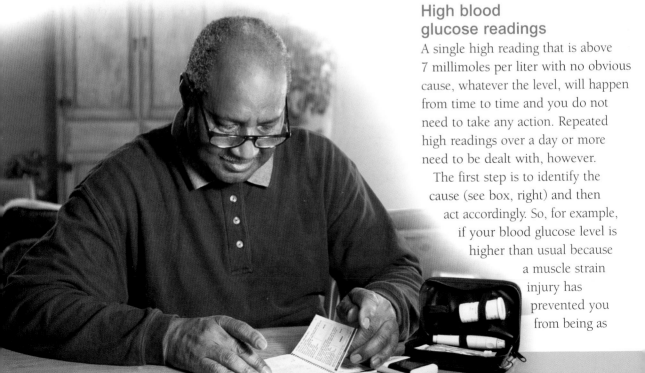

active as usual, you may decide to limit the food you eat or try an alternative activity that doesn't put pressure on the injured muscle.

If stress or illness is causing you to have high readings for a period of longer than one or two days, you can temporarily increase your medication. But remember to return to your usual dose when you are better and your blood glucose level falls. If your weight has increased, you may also need to increase your medication to counteract the insulin resistance this causes.

A high blood glucose level that follows a low blood sugar level, as a result of your hypoglycemic treatment and the extra glucose your body produces, can be prevented only by trying to limit the effect of the hypoglycemic episode as much as possible. This may involve reducing your medication or eating more regularly. In all cases, your blood glucose tests will tell you how successful your actions have been (see pp.110–113 for more on hyperglycemia).

Low blood glucose readings

Blood glucose readings below 4 millimoles per liter should be treated immediately by eating or drinking glucose (see p.106). If you regularly have readings below 4 millimoles per liter, your awareness of the signs of hypoglycemia may be reduced. A hypoglycemic attack can make it difficult for you to think clearly, but once you are feeling

SOME REASONS FOR HIGHS AND LOWS	
An occasional high or low blood glucose level does not indicate that your diabetes is out of control (although a low blood glucose level should always be treated promptly). However, if you notice a pattern of highs or lows, finding out why can help you take corrective action.	
HIGH READINGS	**LOW READINGS**
Having more food than usual or a different type of food. (A specific food may be to blame if it's associated with high readings on several occasions).	Having less food than usual, or taking your insulin or pills and then being unable to eat at the planned time.
Being less physically active than usual.	Being more physically active than usual.
Illness can cause a high blood glucose reading, as can stress hormones.	Stress can make your blood glucose level fall if you respond to it by using up more energy or eating less than usual.
Forgetting to take your pills or your insulin or taking an insufficient dose.	Taking an extra dose of pills, injecting too much insulin, or being on too high a dose of pills or insulin.
Putting on weight.	Losing weight.
Special circumstances, such as a hypoglycemic attack earlier in the day, treated with glucose (when you are hypoglycemic, your liver also converts glycogen into glucose and releases it).	Special circumstances, such as drinking a lot of alcohol without compensating by eating carbohydrate-containing food at the same time or reducing your dosage of medication.

better, determining the cause will help you plan ahead and prevent it from happening again. This might involve reducing your medication, eating more, or altering your activity level.

Whatever course of action you decide to take to prevent a future episode, your tests will tell you how successful you have been. You may need to make several changes to get the levels you want (see pp.102–109 for more on hypoglycemia).

Pills

Controlling your blood glucose level with pills is likely to be part of your daily routine if you have type 2 diabetes. No single pill is right for every person; sometimes you need to try several different pills and doses or take a combination of pills. Whether you are about to start taking pills or have been taking them for some time, it's useful to understand how your particular pills work, have information about dosage, and know of any precautions or contraindications.

Different pills work better for different people— you may need to try more than one pill or different combinations before you find the one that suits you.

Controlling diabetes with pills

Pills are an important way of controlling blood glucose when you have type 2 diabetes. Although the insulin you produce is insufficient or less effective in type 2 diabetes, pills don't actually contain insulin, as it would be broken down during digestion. Instead, pills control your blood glucose in one or more ways.
- Increasing the amount of insulin your body produces.
- Helping your body cells use insulin more efficiently.
- Reducing the amount of glucose your liver produces.
- Slowing down your digestion of carbohydrate-rich foods.

Who needs to take pills?
If you have type 2 diabetes or MODY (see p.16), you will probably need to start taking pills to control your

blood glucose at some point. (If you have type 1 diabetes, you will always need insulin injections rather than pills to control your blood glucose.) If, when you are first diagnosed, your blood glucose level is very high (20 millimoles per liter or more) or you have severe symptoms, you will probably be prescribed pills right away. However, if your blood glucose level is lower than this and you feel well, it is more common for your health professional to recommend that you concentrate on eating a healthy diet, increasing your physical activity, and losing weight if you need to. These measures help reduce the amount of insulin your body needs, so that your own insulin may again be sufficient to effectively control your blood glucose level.

You may be asked to keep your blood glucose level under control in this way for a trial period, usually at least three months, after which your

CONTROLLING BLOOD GLUCOSE WITH PILLS
Pills that are prescribed for diabetes work in various ways to lower your blood glucose level. If you have type 2 diabetes, taking pills, eating healthily, and being physically active are important to keep your diabetes well controlled.

health professional will help you assess how successful this has been. If you need more help to control your diabetes at this or a future assessment, you are prescribed pills. You may manage your diabetes with food, drink, and physical activity for years after diagnosis, or you may need to start taking pills within months.

Being prescribed pills doesn't mean that you have failed to do enough to control your diabetes. It may be because—as is normal in type 2 diabetes—your pancreas gradually produces less and less insulin over time or your body cells have become increasingly resistant to the action of insulin. It is very likely that you will need pills at some point to control type 2 diabetes.

The right pill

Your health professional works with you to decide which pills can best control your diabetes. All pills are prescribed on a trial basis, because it is not until you take a pill that you discover whether it is the right one for you (you may have side effects, for example) and/or is effective. Different pills work better for different people; you may need to try more than one pill or different combinations before you find the one that suits you. Your health professional is likely to recommend an AIC blood test (see pp.66–67) about three months after you have started a new type of pill, in order to assess how well it is controlling your blood glucose level.

A pill that is right for you at one time may not be the one that is right for you permanently. Because type 2 diabetes is a progressive condition in which your insulin production steadily declines, the dose and type of pills you take need to change accordingly. Your health professional may suggest a gradual increase in the

Myth OR TRUTH?

MYTH
If diabetes pills make my blood glucose level normal again, I can stop taking them.

TRUTH
Diabetes pills keep your blood glucose level under control only while you are taking them. If you stop, your blood glucose level rises again. Taking your pills in the right doses and at the right times in relation to food helps keep your blood glucose controlled in the long term.

dose of your pills or may prescribe a different pill or combination of pills. More than 50 percent of people with type 2 diabetes need to start injecting insulin to control their diabetes at some point. How quickly this happens depends on how long your pancreas can produce enough insulin and how long your pills are effective in controlling your blood glucose level.

These are some of the factors that you and your health professional should consider when choosing the right pill for you.

■ **BLOOD GLUCOSE LEVEL** If the pills you are taking aren't controlling your blood glucose level adequately, you may need an increased dose or one or more different types of pill.

■ **YOUR WEIGHT** If you are overweight, pills that cause weight gain would not be the first choice for you.

■ **A PILL'S LENGTH OF ACTION** Some pills work over a long period, others only last a short time. Longer-acting pills need to be taken only once a day, but

> **Q** Can my health professional just keep increasing the dose of my pills each time the pills stop working for me?
>
> **A** All pills work best when you first start taking them. Increasing the dose after this has some effect on your blood glucose level, but it won't have as much effect as the initial dose. (For example, doubling your dose doesn't have double the effect on your blood glucose level.) This is the reason your health professional may sometimes prescribe a new type of pill rather than prescribing the maximum dose of the one you are currently taking.

your chances of a hypoglycemic episode are higher.

■ **YOUR EATING PATTERN** If your lifestyle prevents you from eating regular meals, pills with a short length of action are more appropriate than longer-acting pills.

■ **SIDE EFFECTS** If you experience side effects, you may need a reduced dose or a different type of pill.

Types of pills

Different pills have different actions, doses, and precautions. If you have any concerns about the pills you take, you should consult your health professional. Never exceed the recommended daily dose of pills and don't stop taking them without consulting your health professional first.

Metformin

Metformin (brand name Glucophage) may be the first pill you are prescribed—especially if you are overweight, because it doesn't cause weight gain. Metformin may be prescribed in combination with any of the diabetes pills described here.

■ **HOW THE DRUG WORKS** Even though your pancreas still produces insulin in type 2 diabetes, it doesn't trigger the process by which glucose is taken in by the cells and burned as energy. Metformin counteracts this insulin resistance by increasing your body cells' sensitivity to insulin. It also reduces the amount of glucose that your liver produces.

> If your lifestyle prevents you from eating regular meals, pills with a short length of action are more appropriate than longer-acting pills.

■ **DOSE** Metformin comes in 500mg and 850mg pills. The initial dose is a single pill (500mg) with or after your breakfast or evening meal. This may be increased over time. For example:
• Two pills with or after either your breakfast or evening meal.
• Two pills with or after either your breakfast or evening meal and one pill with or after your lunch.
• Two pills with or after both your breakfast and evening meal.

■ **PRECAUTIONS** The main side effects of metformin are nausea and diarrhea. These are not inevitable, however, and you can reduce the chances of side effects by always taking the pills with or after a meal and by increasing doses gradually. For example, if your health professional prescribes four pills a day, he or she may tell you to build up to this dose by taking one pill a day for the first week, two a day for the second week, until you are having four a day (this may mean that your blood glucose level temporarily remains slightly high) You may need to adjust the dose of metformin for some weeks until you discover the amount that controls your blood glucose without producing side effects. If you have side effects on low doses, you may need a different type of pill. You should not take metformin if you have kidney problems or severe heart disease.

Sulfonylureas

There are a number of different pills in the sulfonylurea group. All work in broadly the same way but have different durations of action. Therefore, some drugs in this group need to be taken more times a day than others. Some commonly prescribed sulfonylureas are gliclazide (Diamicron), glimepiride (Amaryl), and glyburide (Diabeta, Euglucon). Chlorpropamide and tolbutamide are also available but infrequently used.

If you are not overweight, a sulfonylurea may be the first type of pill you are prescribed. A sulfonylurea is sometimes added to your prescription when metformin is no longer controlling your blood glucose level. Other pills for diabetes that may be prescribed in combination with sulfonylureas include rosiglitazone, pioglitazone, acarbose, nateglinide, and repaglinide.

■ **HOW THE DRUGS WORK** A sulfonylurea is an insulin-stimulating pill that works on the beta cells in your pancreas to increase the amount of insulin you produce.

■ **DOSE** The dose is a single pill, which you take just before breakfast. The dose of shorter-acting sulfonylureas may be increased over time to include more than one pill per dose and/or a second dose before your evening meal.

■ **PRECAUTIONS** Side effects of sulfonylureas include weight gain and hypoglycemia. Eating regular meals and snacks can reduce your risk of becoming hypoglycemic. Your health professional can discuss with you how you can best arrange your eating plan if necessary. One sulfonylurea, chlorpropamide, may

Practical tips

REMEMBERING TO TAKE YOUR PILLS

• Every morning, count out your pills for the day; check that you have taken all of them at the end of the day.
• Put the pills in a place that will remind you to take them. For example, in the kitchen.
• As you prepare your meal, also prepare your pills at the same time.
• If necessary, set an alarm for the time you need to take your pills.
• Ask someone to remind you at the time you need to take your pills.
• Always keep a supply of your pills with you in case you are stuck away from home for a period of time.

Side effects
of repaglinide
and nateglinide,
like other insulin-
stimulating
pills such as the
sulfonylureas,
include weight
gain and
hypoglycemia.

cause your face to flush when you drink alcohol and, because it has a longer action than the other pills in the sulfonylurea group, it is also more likely to cause hypoglycemia. For this reason, chlorpropamide is no longer commonly prescribed; however, if you do take it and it works for you, you should continue to take it.

If your liver and kidney function are declining for any reason, your health professional may suggest that you change to a different type of pill. If you are pregnant or breastfeeding, a sulfonylurea would not be recommended.

Some people may experience an adverse interaction between sulfonylureas and drugs such as nonsteroidal anti-inflammatory drugs (NSAIDs) and sulfinpyrazone (which is used to treat rheumatic diseases and gout), chloramphenicol (used to treat ear infections), bosentan (used to treat high blood pressure), and fluconazole and miconazole (used to treat fungal infections).

Thiazolidinediones

Rosiglitazone (brand name Avandia) and pioglitazone (brand name Actos) are the two pills in a group known as thiazolidinediones. They are often referred to by the name glitazones.

Thiazolidinediones can either be prescribed on their own or in combination with another diabetes drug such as metformin or a sulfonylurea.

Q Can I adjust my pill dose myself, or do I have to consult my health professional?

A Because your need for medication is likely to increase over time, and also because of the importance of controlling your blood glucose level when you are ill, you may need to increase the dosage yourself. If you know how your pills work, for how long, and what the maximum dose is, you can make useful adjustments. Regular blood glucose testing will tell you if your adjustments have made a difference. It's also important to inform your physician about any changes you've made.

■ **HOW THE DRUGS WORK**
Thiazolidinediones function by reducing the resistance of your body cells to insulin. They also have a beneficial effect on blood fat levels, which can help protect against cardiovascular disease (see pp.206–211).

■ **DOSE** Pioglitazone is designed to be taken once a day, either one or two pills at a time; rosiglitazone can be taken once or twice a day.

■ **PRECAUTIONS** Side effects of thiazolidinediones include weight gain and retaining extra fluid in your body. You should not take them if you have heart failure or liver problems, if you are pregnant or breastfeeding, or if you are taking pills to get rid of extra fluid in your body. Rarely, some thiazolidinediones have been associated with liver dysfunction; therefore, if you take them, you will need to have a blood test every few months to monitor your liver function.

Repaglinide and Nateglinide

Repaglinide (brand name Prandin) and nateglinide (brand name Starlix) are faster acting than sulfonylureas and less likely to lead to hypoglycemia and weight gain. They are designed to stimulate insulin production for short periods around the times when you eat and are useful if you have a varied daily routine and tend not to eat at regular times. Because they are relatively new, these drugs are less widely prescribed than sulfonylureas. Repaglinide and nateglinide may be prescribed on their own or in combination with metformin.

■ **HOW THE DRUGS WORK** These pills act on the beta cells in your pancreas to help you produce more insulin.

■ **DOSE** Because repaglinide and nateglinide work within a short space of time and their effect wears off quickly, so you need to take one pill before each of your meals. If you miss a meal, you should also skip a pill, otherwise you risk hypoglycemia.

■ **PRECAUTIONS** Side effects of repaglinide and nateglinide, like other insulin-secreting pills such as the sulfonylureas, include weight gain and hypoglycemia. You should not take either repaglinide and nateglinide if you are pregnant or breastfeeding.

Alpha-glucosidase inhibitor

There is one alpha-glucosidase inhibitor: acarbose (brand name Prandase), which blunts the rise in your blood glucose after meals. This drug tends to be prescribed less often because side effects are common.

■ **HOW THE DRUG WORKS** Alpha-glucosidase inhibitor slows down the breakdown of carbohydrate during digestion, so that glucose is released more slowly into your bloodstream. Because your blood glucose level then rises more slowly after a meal, your own insulin can cope better.

■ **DOSE** The initial dose is half or one pill a day with your evening meal (chewed and swallowed with your first mouthful). The dose should be increased slowly, every 2–3 weeks (to avoid side effects), and pills should be split equally between breakfast, lunch, and your evening meal. This gradual increase may mean that your blood glucose level is temporarily high until you find the right dose. The maximum dose is four pills (200mg) three times a day, but side effects may prevent you from reaching this dose.

■ **PRECAUTIONS** The main effect of an alpha-glucosidase inhibitor is on your bowel: it can cause flatulence and diarrhea. If these are severe, you may need a different type of pill; consult your health professional before you stop taking this drug. You should not take acarbose if you are pregnant or breastfeeding.

PILLS AND MEALTIMES
Taking your pills at the right time in relation to your meal, before, with, or after eating, will maximize their effectiveness in controlling your blood glucose level.

Insulin

Insulin is essential if you have type 1 diabetes and is likely to be part of your treatment at some point if you have type 2 diabetes. There are many types and regimens of insulin and these can be adapted and the doses adjusted to help you get the best control of your diabetes. Knowing about the different delivery devices available—and how to use them—can help you find one to suit you. New forms of insulin delivery may be on the way; alternatives to injections are always being researched.

Controlling diabetes with insulin

Insulin is an essential hormone; without it your body cells cannot take in glucose from your blood to use for energy. This leaves you with little energy and gives rise to other symptoms of diabetes (see pp.18–19). It also forces your body to find alternative sources of energy, such as body fat (see p.113).

If your pancreas no longer produces insulin, or if it produces so little that the pills you take for diabetes are no longer effective, you need an external source of insulin, usually in the form of regular injections. Some people receive insulin continuously through a device called an insulin pump. You may be daunted by the idea of injecting insulin, but if you do need it, the many types, doses, and ways of injecting insulin that are available will allow you and your

health professional to match your treatment closely to your needs. The goal of insulin treatment is to enable you to feel well on a day-to-day basis and to reduce your risk of long-term complications.

Your insulin regimen (see pp.87–90), will need to change from time to time to make sure that it controls your blood glucose level effectively and matches your lifestyle.

Who needs insulin?

If you have type 1 diabetes, you don't produce any insulin and your life depends on receiving insulin by injection or insulin pump. If you have type 2 diabetes or MODY (see p.16) and your blood glucose level reaches the point at which it can no longer be controlled by pills (see pp.76–81), you will also be prescribed insulin. If you have type 2 diabetes or MODY, you may occasionally need insulin on

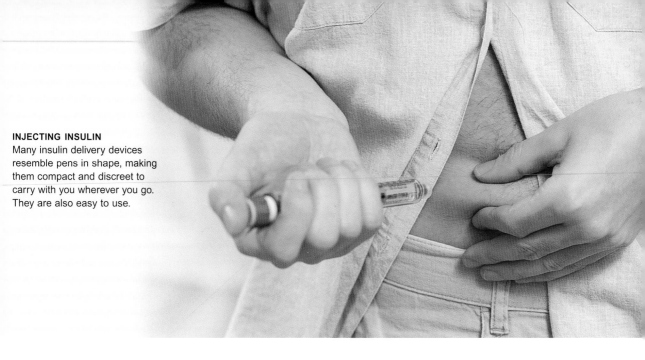

INJECTING INSULIN
Many insulin delivery devices resemble pens in shape, making them compact and discreet to carry with you wherever you go. They are also easy to use.

a temporary basis, for example, if you go into the hospital for major surgery, have a heart attack or another serious illness, and you are too ill to eat and drink. In these situations, insulin is given by infusion (see pp.134–135) and you may need to continue injecting it after leaving the hospital.

If you have gestational diabetes (see pp.144–145), and changes to your food intake and activity level do not control your blood glucose level, you will need insulin treatment until the end of your pregnancy. You also need insulin during your pregnancy if you had diabetes that was treated with pills, because diabetes pills are not recommended during pregnancy and when you are breastfeeding.

How insulin controls blood glucose

The insulin you receive by injection or pump works in the same way as the insulin produced in the pancreas of a person who doesn't have diabetes. It lowers the level of glucose in your blood by enabling your body cells to take in glucose, and your liver and muscles to store glucose in the form of glycogen. Insulin also plays an important part in preventing glycogen from being converted back into glucose. This keeps your blood glucose level from rising unnecessarily. Your insulin treatment is designed to mimic the natural way insulin is released in your body, which is to rise and fall according to the level of glucose in your blood.

Insulin strength and doses

Insulin is measured in International Units, or "units" for short. There are 100 units to every milliliter (mL). Insulin usually comes in either a small 10mL (1,000-unit) glass bottle, a 3mL (300-unit) cartridge, or a 3mL (300-unit) delivery device. Unlike other forms of medication, such as

The insulin you receive by injection or pump works in the same way as the insulin produced in the pancreas of a person who doesn't have diabetes.

**INSULIN PRODUCTION IN
A HEALTHY BODY**
The pancreas maintains a
background level of insulin and
produces extra insulin to deal
with rises in blood glucose after
eating and drinking.

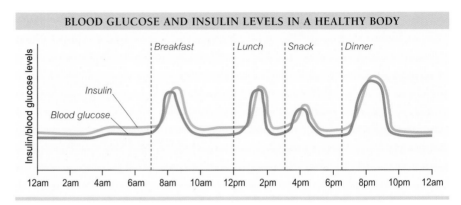

BLOOD GLUCOSE AND INSULIN LEVELS IN A HEALTHY BODY

painkillers or antibiotics, there is no universal maximum dose of insulin. Everyone's needs are different and your insulin dose will be tailored to your needs. You will usually start on a small dose (10–20 units per day) of insulin and increase or decrease this to keep your fasting blood glucose level between 4 and 7 millimoles per liter. The amount of insulin you need to keep your blood glucose level within the recommended range will vary according to different circumstances (see pp.93–95).

Types of insulin

If you need insulin to control your diabetes, you will be prescribed one or more of five main types. The difference between each type is the length of time it works in your body after you have injected it. You might find that one type of insulin always suits you, or you may need to change types or use different combinations from time to time.

Most insulin used today is "human insulin," which means that it has been manufactured in a laboratory to work in a similar way to the insulin produced by a healthy human pancreas. If you have had diabetes for many years, you may still take animal insulin, which is produced from the pancreas of a pig. However, animal insulin, which is not available in a rapid-acting form, is less commonly used and is no longer prescribed as a first choice of insulin.

Rapid-acting insulin analogue

Rapid-acting insulin first became available during the late 1990s. It is also known as insulin analogue, which means that it is made by altering the structure of insulin so that it starts working within 5 minutes after you have injected it.

Because it begins to work so quickly, you can inject rapid-acting insulin analogue just before you eat or up to 15 minutes after you have eaten. This can be useful when you don't know exactly when your food will arrive or how much there will be. Another advantage of taking rapid-acting insulin analogue is that you can decide how much insulin you need in relation to the quantity of food you are eating.

Once rapid-acting insulin analogue is in your bloodstream, it reaches peak action after 1–2 hours and wears off after 4 hours, approximately the time that is needed to deal with the rise in blood glucose resulting from your meal. This short duration decreases the likelihood of hypoglycemia between meals.

However, once rapid-acting insulin analogue starts to wear off, your blood glucose level rises. This means that you also need to take an intermediate or longer-acting insulin. You can mix the two insulins yourself (except glargine), use a pre-mixed insulin, or take them separately.

Rapid-acting insulin analogue can also be given as a single injection for an unexpectedly high blood glucose level, caused by illness or stress, for example. If you have an insulin pump, you are likely to use rapid-acting insulin analogue. Rapid-acting insulin analogue can be used by both children and adults, and there is no evidence to suggest that it shouldn't be used during pregnancy.

> **Q** Why do fast-acting insulins tend to be clear and longer-acting insulins tend to be cloudy?
>
> **A** Fast-acting insulins are naturally clear. Most longer-acting insulins are simply shorter-acting insulins that have had protamine and/or zinc added to them to make them last longer. These substances make the insulin appear cloudy. However, insulin glargine, which is an extended long-acting insulin analogue, is clear.

Fast-acting insulin

This is also called soluble insulin and is a clear solution that takes about 30 minutes to start working after you have injected it. For this reason, you need to leave a gap of 20–30 minutes between injecting your insulin and starting to eat. Once fast-acting insulin is in your bloodstream, it reaches a peak of action after 2–4 hours and can keep working for up to 8 hours before gradually wearing off.

Because fast-acting insulin works for several hours, you may need to balance its action by eating some carbohydrate-containing food as a snack 2–3 hours after a meal—this prevents your blood glucose level

Because fast-acting insulin wears off after a relatively short period of time, you also need some longer-acting insulin to make sure that you have insulin available throughout the day and night.

INSULIN ACTION TIMES

Rapid-acting Fast-acting Long-acting Intermediate-acting Extended long-acting

Insulin level

Hours
0 2 4 6 8 10 12 14 16 18 20 22 24

DURATION OF ACTION
Rapid- and fast-acting insulins begin working quickly, and have a relatively short action time—boosting your insulin level to deal with mealtimes. Intermediate-, long-, and extended long-acting insulin analogues have much longer action times, providing a background level of insulin. You may need one type of insulin or more than one type to control your blood glucose level.

from falling below 4 millimoles per liter and making you hypoglycemic (see pp.102–109). Because fast-acting insulin wears off after a relatively short period of time, you also need some intermediate or longer-acting insulin to make sure that you have insulin available throughout the day and night. You can mix fast-acting and intermediate or longer-acting insulin yourself or you can use a pre-mixed insulin. You can also take fast-acting insulin at mealtimes and a longer-acting insulin at bedtime and/or in the morning.

If your blood glucose level becomes very high, due to illness or stress, for example, you may be taught to correct this by taking an extra dose of fast-acting insulin. Fast-acting insulin is the type of insulin commonly used in hospital insulin infusions and can be used by people of any age or in any circumstances.

Intermediate-acting insulin

This is also called isophane or NPH insulin and is cloudy rather than clear. It is made by adding substances to shorter-acting insulin to make it work longer—up to about 18 hours. It reaches a peak of action between 4 and 8 hours. This helps control your blood glucose level throughout the day, but you may need to eat something around the time of the peak of action to prevent hypoglycemia. If you have type 1 diabetes, you may be prescribed an intermediate-acting insulin with a fast-acting insulin to

THE EFFECTS OF DIFFERENT TYPES OF INSULIN

Your health professional prescribes one or more insulins to match your individual medical and practical needs. It's important to understand when different injections of insulin have an effect on your blood glucose level to help you decide when blood glucose tests will be most useful.

TYPE OF INSULIN	ONSET	PEAK	DURATION
Rapid-acting analogue (clear): Humalog® (insulin lispro) Novorapid® (insulin aspart)	10–15 minutes	60–90 minutes	4–5 hours
Fast-acting (clear): Humulin® -R, Novolin®ge Toronto	30 minutes to 1 hour	2–4 hours	5–8 hours
Intermediate-acting (cloudy): Humulin® -N, Humulin® -L, Novolin®ge NPH	1–3 hours	5–8 hours	Up to 18 hours
Long-acting (cloudy): Humulin® -U	3–4 hours	8–15 hours	22–26 hours
Extended long-acting analogue: Lantus® (insulin glargine)	90 minutes	N/A	24 hours
Premixed (cloudy): Humalog® Mix25™, Humulin® (20/80, 30/70), Novolin®ge (10.90, 20/80, 30/70, 40/60, 50/50), NovoRapid Mix®	N/A	N/A	N/A

Note: A single vial contains a fixed ratio of insulin (% rapid- or fast-acting to % intermediate-acting insulin)

keep your blood glucose level from rising after your fast-acting insulin has worn off. If you have type 2 diabetes, you may be prescribed intermediate-acting insulin on its own, or in combination with a fast-acting insulin or pills (see pp.76–81).

Long-acting insulin

Long-acting insulin starts to work after 3 hours, reaches a peak of action between 8 and 15 hours, and is effective for up to 24 hours. You may need to eat something when it is at its peak to avoid hypoglycemia.

If you have type 1 diabetes, you may combine long-acting insulin with a fast-acting insulin for insulin over a 24-hour period and to keep your blood glucose level from rising too high after meals. If you have type 2 diabetes, you may use long-acting insulin on its own, or in combination with a fast-acting insulin or pills (see pp.76–81).

Extended long-acting insulin analogue

Extended long-acting insulin analogue, also called glargine (lantus), is a new kind of long-acting insulin with no peak of action. It starts working within 90 minutes and is effective for about 24 hours. With no peak of action, you are less likely to experience hypoglycemia than with other long-acting insulins.

If you have type 1 diabetes, you may be prescribed an extended long-acting insulin analogue in combination with rapid-acting insulin analogue given separately at mealtimes. (You can't mix extended long-acting insulin analogue with another insulin in a syringe.) For type 2 diabetes, you may be prescribed extended long-acting insulin analogue on its own, or combined with rapid-acting insulin analogue or pills (see pp.76–81).

Insulin regimens

The amount of insulin you need a day and the type or combination of insulin types you use is known as an insulin regimen. Which regimen is best for you depends on the type of diabetes you have and your daily routine.

The regimen prescribed for you when you are diagnosed with type 1 diabetes or when you start insulin with type 2 diabetes, is unlikely to be the regimen that works for you permanently. Lifestyle changes, such as a new job or a major illness, can significantly alter your insulin needs. Your health professional works with you to decide on the regimen that best controls your diabetes in your particular circumstances.

The regimen prescribed for you when you are diagnosed with type 1 diabetes or when you start insulin with type 2 diabetes, is unlikely to be the regimen that works for you permanently.

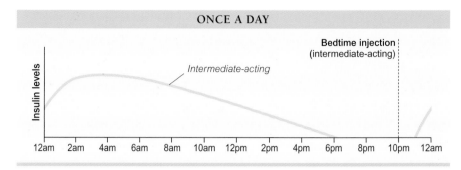

ONCE A DAY

Bedtime injection
(intermediate-acting)

Intermediate-acting

If you have type 2 diabetes, you may progress from a once-a-day to a twice-a-day regimen if the former does not adequately control your blood glucose level.

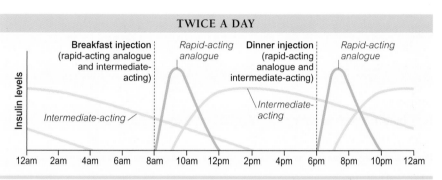

TWICE A DAY

Breakfast injection
(rapid-acting analogue
and intermediate-
acting)

Rapid-acting
analogue

Dinner injection
(rapid-acting
analogue and
intermediate-acting)

Rapid-acting
analogue

Intermediate-acting

Intermediate-
acting

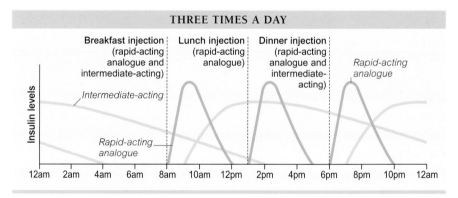

THREE TIMES A DAY

Breakfast injection
(rapid-acting
analogue and
intermediate-acting)

Lunch injection
(rapid-acting
analogue)

Dinner injection
(rapid-acting
analogue and
intermediate-
acting)

Rapid-acting
analogue

Intermediate-acting

Rapid-acting
analogue

FOUR TIMES A DAY

Breakfast injection
(rapid-acting
analogue)

Lunch injection
(rapid-acting
analogue)

Dinner injection
(rapid-acting
analogue)

Bedtime
injection
(extended
long-acting
analogue)

Rapid-
acting
analogue

Extended
long-acting
analogue

COMMON INSULIN REGIMENS
These are the most common insulin combinations for each of the insulin regimens. Each regimen provides a background level of insulin and the twice-, three-times-, and four-times-a-day regimens give extra boosts of insulin when needed.

Once a day

If you have type 2 diabetes and you need to take insulin as well as pills, you are likely to start with one injection a day to cover the rise in blood glucose after meals and in the morning. If you have type 1 diabetes, you would not be prescribed a once-a-day regimen because this would not give you enough insulin to cover your mealtimes.

The insulin prescribed for a once-a-day regimen is an intermediate-, a peakless long-acting or, rarely, a long-acting insulin. You can inject it at bedtime to avoid morning hyperglycemia caused by the release of glucose into the blood from the liver during the night. One advantage of bedtime injections is that you don't have to remember to carry injecting equipment with you during the day. However, if your lifestyle demands it—if you work night shifts, for example—you can inject insulin in the morning. Another advantage of a once-a-day regimen is that weight gain and hypoglycemia are less common than with other regimens.

Twice a day

If you have type 2 diabetes, you may progress from a once-a-day to a twice-a-day regimen if the former does not adequately control your blood glucose level. You may also be on a twice-a-day-regimen if you have type 1 diabetes. You may be prescribed one of the following types or combinations of insulin to take twice a day:

- Either an intermediate- or, rarely, a long-acting insulin.
- An intermediate- or, rarely, long-acting insulin that comes ready-mixed with a rapid- or fast-acting insulin.
- An intermediate- or, rarely, long-acting insulin that you mix yourself with a rapid- or fast-acting insulin.

Whichever of these three options you are prescribed, they are designed so that you inject yourself once in the morning, before or just after breakfast, to control your blood glucose level during the day, and once again in the evening, either before or after your evening meal or before you go to bed, to control your blood glucose level during the night. If your twice-a-day regimen contains rapid- or fast-acting insulin, you will need to take it in relation to mealtimes. You need to eat regularly on a twice-a-day regimen to prevent hypoglycemia.

Three times a day

If you find that there are still times when your blood glucose level is too high when you are on a twice-a-day regimen, you may be prescribed a third dose of rapid- or fast-acting insulin, usually at lunchtime or with your evening meal, depending on the timing of your intermediate-acting insulin.

A three-times-a-day regimen may suit you in the long term or you may only need a third dose of insulin temporarily—for example, if your work or social life has changed recently or if you are recovering from an illness.

Myth OR TRUTH?

MYTH
The longer you have diabetes, the more daily injections you need.

TRUTH
The type and regimen of insulin that you have is not dependent on how long you have had diabetes. It is very likely that from time to time you will need to change the number of injections you have as a result of changes in your life. For example, you may become pregnant or start a new job. If you start to develop long-term complications, you may also need more frequent insulin injections in order to improve your blood glucose control. These changes could be required at any stage after you start to take insulin.

Four times a day or more (basal bolus)

This is also known as a multiple injection regimen. The goal is to replicate as closely as possible the normal rising and falling insulin levels of a person who does not have diabetes. One dose of extended long-acting insulin analogue in the morning, evening, or at bedtime, or one or two doses of intermediate, provides a background (known as basal) level of insulin throughout the day. This is supplemented by booster doses of rapid-acting insulin (known as boluses) taken at mealtimes to match the carbohydrate in the meal. Whether you take it before, during, or after the meal depends on your blood sugar level before the meal.

A four-times-a-day regimen can help you match the amount of insulin you need to the amount of food you are eating at that time. This helps you avoid a hypoglycemic response during meals and reduces the number of snacks you need. The longer-acting insulin helps keep your blood glucose level within a healthy range between the times at which your rapid-acting insulin has finished working.

Another advantage of the four-times-a-day regimen is that you can make immediate adjustments to your bolus doses based on your activity levels, your food intake, and the results of your blood glucose tests. You can also give extra boluses in certain situations, such as when you are ill or having larger meals or more snacks than usual.

Continuous delivery

The alternative to single or multiple insulin injections every day is to take it continuously by means of a pump (see pp.96–97). A pump constantly delivers a basal rate of rapid-acting insulin analogue into your body via a tube in your abdomen and delivers extra doses, called boluses, at mealtimes and when your blood glucose is high.

Adjusting doses of insulin

An important aspect of diabetes control is adjusting or fine-tuning your dose of insulin to prevent or compensate for high or low blood glucose levels. Just as the healthy pancreas secretes differing amounts of insulin according to the level of glucose in the blood, you may need to inject differing amounts of insulin based on what and how much you eat, how active you are, and based on the results of your blood glucose tests. (These results will reflect your food intake and activity as well as other factors, such as illness and stress.)

How often you adjust your insulin dose depends on your regimen and on how well your diabetes is controlled. You may make daily or weekly adjustments over a period of time, or you may only need to make adjustments in special circumstances, such as vacations or when you are ill. When you first start insulin treatment, you are likely to receive frequent advice on dosages from your health

---

Practical tips

ADJUSTING YOUR INSULIN DOSE

- If you take a combination of insulins, adjusting the insulin that is working at the time of your high/low blood glucose test results will have an effect at the time you want it to.

- A dose change that works for someone else will not necessarily work for you. Insulin dose changes affect everybody differently. It takes practice to become confident about managing dose changes.

A MONITORING DIARY—USING A FOUR-TIMES-A-DAY REGIMEN

Day	Breakfast rapid-acting	Lunch rapid-acting	Dinner rapid-acting	Bedtime intermediate	Before breakfast	2 hours after breakfast	Before lunch	2 hours after lunch	Before evening meal	2 hours after evening meal	Before bed	During night	Notes/Action
	Rapid-/intermediate-acting insulin injection time and dose				Blood glucose level (millimoles per liter)								
Mon	6v	6v	10v	20v	7.0	–	14.5	–	10.1	–	6.8	–	BG too high during day. Count breakfast carbs. Test tomorrow.
Tue	6v	6v	10v	20v	7.2	–	14.8	–	9.8	–	6.5	–	Increase morning rapid-acting by 2v tomorrow.
Wed	8v	6v	14v	20v	7.6	–	7.2	–	15.3	–	8.2	–	Extra insulin (out for dinner in the evening).
Thu	8v	6v	10v	20v	7.4	–	7.1	8.2	15.9	–	8.0	–	BG too high before dinner/bedtime. Count lunch carbs. Increase lunchtime rapid-acting by 2v.
Fri	8v	8v	10v	20v	8.5	–	7.1	–	12.8	–	6.2	–	Morning BG too high – increase lunchtime insulin again.
Sat	8v	10v	10v	22v	8.8	–	7.0	–	7.6	–	6.4	–	Morning BG still too high. Increase evening intermediate.
Sun	8v	10v	10v	22v	3.8	3.0	6.8	–	7.6	–	5.0	–	Hypoglycemic this morning; alcohol last night? Reduce bedtime insulin tomorrow if it happens again.

professional, based on your blood glucose test results. Over time, you'll learn to make your own adjustments.

General guidelines

If your home blood glucose tests reveal a pattern of results outside the healthy range (4–7 millimoles per liter), you need to consider which aspect of your diabetes management is responsible. For example, have you been eating more or less food or been more or less active than usual? If you can

modify some aspect of your daily routine to bring your blood glucose test results back into a healthy range, this might be your first course of action. If you can't do this or it doesn't give you the results you need, consider adjusting your insulin dose. The following guidelines apply to changing insulin doses:
• In general, avoid changing your insulin dose in response to a single test result. Instead, base changes on patterns in your results.

ADJUSTING INSULIN DOSES
Making changes to your insulin in relation to your blood glucose test results is an important part of keeping your diabetes under control. This example of a personal chart shows a regimen of mealtime rapid- and bedtime intermediate-acting insulin.

MYTH
I have to stay on the insulin regimen I've always had.

TRUTH
There are lots of insulin regimens. The right one for you keeps your diabetes well controlled but also fits in with your lifestyle. From time to time, you may need to change your regimen to match changes in your daily routine.

- If your blood glucose level is high for more than a day or two, and other measures aren't working, you need more insulin.
- If your blood glucose level is low for more than a day or two, for no apparent reason, you need less insulin.
- Start by increasing or decreasing your insulin dose by 2–4 units at a time. If you usually take large doses of insulin, 40–60 units in a single dose, for example, you may need larger dose changes to have an effect—talk to your health professional.
- If you inject insulin more than once a day, change only one insulin dose at a time. If you change more than one dose, the effect may be unclear and you may end up with too much or too little insulin in your system.
- Use your blood glucose test results to indicate if your change has worked.
- If you are on a twice-a-day regimen with long-acting insulin, wait at least a day before making further dose changes—this insulin stays in the body for up to 24 hours, so you need this amount of time to assess whether your dose change has worked.
- Children generally need smaller dose changes. For example, 1 unit, or even half a unit, at a time will be effective.

Adjusting a once-a-day dose

With this regimen, you can decide whether to increase or decrease your insulin dose depending on too low or too high a blood glucose level. You can assess this by testing your blood glucose level at different times of the day—for example, when you get up in the morning, before or two hours after your lunch, and before or two hours after your evening meal. If you change your dose and it hasn't brought your blood glucose level under control, consider making a further dose change in a day or two.

Adjusting a twice-a-day dose

If you take intermediate- or long-acting insulin by itself, or intermediate- or long-acting insulin that is ready mixed with a fast- or rapid-acting insulin, you need to decide which of your two injections—morning or evening—you need to adjust. If you want to exert greater control over your blood glucose level before lunch, in the afternoon, and before your evening meal, you should adjust the dose of your morning injection of insulin. If, on the other hand, you want to exert greater control over your blood glucose level in the evening, overnight, and first thing in the morning, you should adjust the dose of your evening injection.

If you inject twice a day and you mix your own rapid- or fast-acting and intermediate- or long-acting insulin, you can adjust only the rapid- or fast-acting or only the longer-acting insulin, depending on the time of day your blood glucose level is rising or falling. You should see the results of your changes at that time the next day. If the changes have not achieved a blood glucose level of 4–7 millimoles per liter, consider making a further change.

Adjusting a three- or four-times-a-day dose

Three- and four-times-a-day regimens are designed to enable you to make frequent adjustments to your dose of rapid- or fast-acting insulin at mealtimes as well as changes to your longer-acting insulin. With rapid-acting insulin in particular, you can do this according to the size and type of meal you are about to eat—more or less carbohydrate in your meal means you need to inject more or less insulin. If you do not know how much you will eat, you can inject your rapid-acting insulin after you have eaten. You can measure the effect of your dose change by testing your blood glucose two hours later.

If you use fast-acting insulin and change the dose of your breakfast injection, you need to be aware that it affects your blood glucose level not just two hours after eating, but up until lunchtime. Similarly, a change in your lunchtime dose continues to affect your blood glucose level in the late afternoon. So, for example, an increased dose might make a hypoglycemic reaction more likely 4–6 hours later, even though it corrects a high blood glucose level after 2 hours.

If you notice that your blood glucose level is high or low between meals or first thing in the morning, even though you have been changing the dose of your mealtime insulin injections, you may need to change your longer-acting insulin dose. Monitor your blood glucose level several times over the day to assess the effect of such a change because it is working throughout this period.

Dealing with different situations

If you are aware of situations that are likely to significantly raise or lower your blood glucose level, take action to prevent this from happening.

■ **EATING OUT** If you are going out for a meal or know that you are going to be eating a lot of extra food on a particular occasion, you can prevent your blood glucose level from rising too high by increasing your dose of insulin before you eat. Alternatively, if you use rapid-acting insulin, you can take insulin after you have eaten and base the dose on the type and size of your meal. When you increase your insulin dose, work out how long the insulin will stay in your body and when it will have its peak effect (see p.85), since you may need to have a snack at this point to avoid hypoglycemia. Also, bear in mind that regularly taking extra insulin to cope with extra food consumption can lead to weight gain. See pp.30–43 for healthy eating guidelines.

> When you increase your insulin dose, work out how long the insulin will stay in your body and when it will have its peak effect.

My experience

"I had to try various regimens before I could control my blood glucose without hypoglycemia— 6 different regimens in 20 years!" STUART

COMMENT Adjusting your doses of insulin in response to your blood glucose level can help keep your diabetes well controlled, but sometimes a change of regimen might give you even more flexibility and control. Your health professional will be able to advise you.

■ **PHYSICAL ACTIVITY** Your blood glucose level falls in response to physical activity so, if you are going to be more active than usual, you may need to decrease your insulin dose so that you don't become hypoglycemic or have to eat more to counteract a low blood glucose level. For example, if you are going swimming during the morning, you could decrease your morning dose of insulin. Any kind of activity can lower your blood glucose level; dog walking and having sex, for example, are both forms of physical activity.

■ **ILLNESS** A rise in blood glucose is a normal part of your body's response to illness. This happens even if you are not eating, and it can increase the likelihood of additional infections, a slow recovery time, diabetic ketoacidosis if you have type 1 diabetes, and hyperosmolar non-ketotic coma if you have type 2 diabetes. For this reason, it is important to increase your insulin dose by as much as necessary (based on information from frequent blood glucose tests) to keep your glucose level to at most 10 millimoles per liter. During illness, this increase may be 2–4 units or more at each dose. Alternatively, your health professional may recommend more frequent injections.

As you recover, your blood glucose level usually falls and you will need to reduce your insulin again. Or you may find that your blood glucose level remains high as your body recovers from illness (see pp.130–133).

■ **FASTING** If you are otherwise well and fasting, whether in preparation for a medical investigation or for religious or other reasons, you will need to decrease your insulin dose. If you have type 1 diabetes, you need a lower-than-usual dose of insulin for the duration of your fast. If you have type 2 diabetes, you may be able to have a greatly reduced insulin dose or even stop insulin altogether while you are fasting (because you may still be able to produce some insulin yourself).

If you are not fasting completely but are giving up some types of food, you need to tailor your insulin regimen so that you receive enough insulin when you eat, but not so much that you become hypoglycemic at other times. A basal-bolus regimen using a rapid-acting insulin analogue may be useful; ask your health professional.

If you need to fast for a morning medical investigation, you can decrease your insulin dose on the

Myth OR TRUTH?

MYTH
When you inject insulin, it goes into a vein.

TRUTH
The insulin you inject yourself doesn't go directly into your bloodstream. Instead, the needle goes into the subcutaneous fat layer (underneath your skin) and the insulin gets absorbed from here into your bloodstream. If you use the correct injection technique, you will not inject into a vein by accident. Sometimes, if you are in the hospital, you might be attached to an infusion of insulin that goes directly into your vein, but this is temporary and you would never need to do this yourself at home.

Dosage dial

Side plunger, easier for small or arthritic hands

Replaceable insulin cartridge

Attachable needle

Side-grip plunger device (reusable)

Dosage dial and plunger

Bright colors and pattern appeal to young children

Pen top coverin attachable nee

Child's device (reusable)

evening before the investigation and, if you usually have insulin in the morning, delay this until after the investigation, when you are able to eat again. If you need further information about fasting, ask your health professional.

Insulin equipment

There is a wide variety of equipment designed to deliver insulin. Some people prefer to inject insulin using a needle and syringe; most prefer the convenience of an injection device and insulin cartridge. Receiving insulin continuously via a pump is another alternative. The injection equipment you are offered depends on the type and brand of insulin you are taking, as well as your insulin regimen.

■ **INJECTION DEVICES WITH ATTACHABLE NEEDLES** These devices hold 300 units of insulin and consist of a plunger, a dose-dialing system, and an

Q **What can I do if I am scared of needles?**

A Being scared of injecting before you have ever tried it is common, but true needle phobia is very rare. You may have visions of having to use large needles or inject into a vein. Neither is the case when you are injecting insulin. Try inserting an insulin needle under your skin with your health professional's guidance. You may find this easier and less painful than you expected. This will help prepare you for giving yourself injections on a daily basis. If you are really phobic, jet injectors, which do not have needles, are available on prescription.

attachable needle. They are a convenient and discreet way to inject insulin. Most devices are pen-shaped and come in either reusable or disposable forms. Reusable insulin devices contain cartridges of insulin that you can remove and replace when they are empty. Disposable insulin devices contain an integral insulin

INSULIN DEVICES
Reusable devices have a replaceable insulin cartridge, or they draw insulin from a bottle. Disposable devices are pre-filled with insulin. All types use a needle, except for the jet injector, which fires a stream of insulin through the skin under pressure.

Plunger — Plunger
Electronic memory displays last dose taken
Replaceable insulin cartridge
Dosage dial
Attachable needle

Electronic memory device (reusable)

Plunger
Dosage display
Insulin integral cartridge
Compartment of insulin
Attachable needle

Fixed-dose device (disposable)

Plunger
0 5
50 10
45 15
40 20
35 30 25
Easy dial for arthritic hands, and easy-to-see numbers
Integral insulin cartridge
Attachable needle

Easy dial device (disposable)

Plunger
Insulin is drawn into the syringe from a bottle
Integral needle

Syringe (disposable)

Insulin is drawn into injector from a bottle
Jet nozzle

Jet injector device (reusable)

REUSABLE INSULIN DEVICE
Devices such as this one use insulin cartridges, which are inserted into a holder, and have a dose-dialing system and a plunger. A new needle is attached each time it is used.

Cap | Needle with protective cover | Cartridge holder | Insulin cartridge

cartridge and are thrown away when the insulin runs out—they may last a few days or weeks, depending on how much insulin you take. Whether you have a reusable or disposable device depends on your lifestyle and the brand of insulin you use.

A needle must be fitted to any type of insulin device before use and disposed of afterward. Needles come in four lengths: 5mm, 6mm, 8mm, and 12.7mm. Which length of needle you use depends on which is most comfortable, and on the depth of the fat layer under your skin. The less fat you have, the shorter the needle you will need—children normally require shorter-length needles, for example.

If a needle is too long, you may inject into your muscle. In that case, insulin will reach your bloodstream more quickly and cause your blood glucose level to vary unpredictably (see p.98).

■ **SYRINGES WITH NEEDLES** A traditional syringe holds up to 30, 50, or 100 units of insulin and comes with an 8mm- or 12.7mm-long needle already attached. A syringe and needle is smaller than other devices, but you need to draw up your insulin from a bottle each time you inject. This may be less convenient if you need to inject when you are out.

■ **NEEDLE-FREE JET INJECTOR** This device sends a fine stream of insulin through your skin under pressure, removing the necessity to insert a needle into your body. If you are scared of needles, this device may be of use, although it is larger than most. As with syringes, you need to draw up your insulin from a bottle each time you need a dose.

■ **INSULIN PUMP** A small electronic device that you wear all the time, an insulin pump delivers a basal dose of insulin constantly through a fine tube. The tube, which needs to be changed every two or three days, is connected to your body—usually your abdomen—through a needle or small plastic tube. The pump contains a syringeful or a cartridge of rapid- or fast-acting insulin. To deliver extra doses of insulin (boluses)—at each mealtime, for example—you press a button. If your blood glucose level falls, due to physical activity, for example, you can program the pump

INSULIN PUMP
An insulin pump delivers insulin continuously through a fine tube into your abdomen through a tiny needle. Pumps can offer good control of blood glucose combined with greater freedom about what and when you eat.

*Dosage dial
and plunger*

Dose reading

to deliver less insulin. An insulin pump keeps a record of the doses you have received and when. It can be kept inside your pocket or can be attached to your belt or clothes. Some pumps are waterproof, and you can take off a non-waterproof pump for a short time to bathe or go swimming. If a pump isn't working properly or the insulin is running out, the device will set off an alarm.

Choosing your injection site

Insulin is injected into the fat layer under your skin. The most common injection sites are your thighs, buttocks, or abdomen; your subcutaneous fat layer is too thin in other parts of your body.

Q **What would happen if I accidentally injected my insulin into a muscle?**

A Insulin would get into your bloodstream more quickly than usual, so you may find that your blood glucose level also falls more quickly. In this situation, you may be more likely to have a hypoglycemic reaction. Sometimes, unknowingly injecting into muscle may cause fluctuations in blood glucose. Using a shorter needle or a pinch-up technique (see p.98) can help you inject insulin correctly into the subcutaneous fat layer.

Whichever site you choose to inject into, it is important to change the site frequently. If you repeatedly inject into one site, the frequent exposure to insulin affects your fat cells and causes the area to become lumpy and hard (see lipohypertrophy, pp.212–213).

Although injecting into a lumpy site may be more comfortable than injecting into a non-lumpy site because the skin there has lost sensitivity, this isn't recommended because insulin will enter your bloodstream less efficiently, making it difficult for you to control your blood glucose level. Try to vary injection sites by injecting into your abdomen for a few days, followed by your thighs and then your buttocks. Even if you prefer to inject one of these sites more than others, make sure that you inject over a wide area within that site rather than restricting all your injections to one small place.

When choosing an injection site, you need to take into account the fact that insulin is absorbed into your bloodstream at slightly different speeds from different sites—fastest from your abdomen and slowest from your buttocks. Insulin also works more quickly if you use the muscles near the injection site vigorously soon after you have injected—for example, if you inject into your thigh and then go bicycling. The activity means that insulin circulates much faster than if you injected into a different site.

Front

Back

INJECTION SITES
Knowing where on your body to inject your insulin is important. The colored areas on these diagrams are sites that can be used for injections. You need to change injection sites regularly in order to avoid skin problems.

HOW TO USE AN INSULIN DEVICE

Most insulin devices, whether reusable or disposable, work in the same way, although the details may vary slightly from one device to another—consult the manufacturer's instructions if you are in doubt. Check the appearance and expiration date of your insulin before you inject yourself (see right). This person is using the pinch-up technique (see right).

1 Pull off the outer cover of your insulin device and screw a needle into the cartridge in its holder. Remove the needle's inner cap.

2 If you are injecting a cloudy insulin, invert your device so that it is uniformly cloudy. Dial a small dose of 2–4 units and press the plunger until a drop of insulin appears at the end of the needle (this is called an air shot).

3 Dial the dose that you wish to inject. Then, pinch up a fold of skin at your chosen injection site (in this case the abdomen). Insert the needle into the pinched-up skin, making sure the insulin device is at a 90-degree angle to your body.

4 Press the plunger and keep it depressed while you inject your dose of insulin. Then, leave the needle in your skin for about 10 seconds before you remove it. Dispose of your needle if you need to and replace the cap of your device.

How to inject yourself

Preparing your insulin and using the correct technique to inject is important to enable insulin to work effectively. The precise process of giving yourself an injection depends on whether you are using an insulin device (see box, left), or a syringe (see box, right). Before you inject you need to check your insulin and decide which injection technique you are going to use.

Checking your insulin

Before you inject insulin, check its appearance and expiration date. If it is cloudy when it is meant to be clear, it has a pink tinge, looks lumpy, or contains particles even after gentle rotation, discard it and use a new bottle, cartridge, or disposable device.

Injection techniques

You may have been taught one of two injection techniques.

■ **PINCH-UP TECHNIQUE** This technique involves pinching your skin and subcutaneous fat between your thumb and index finger. Once you have "pinched up," you insert your needle at an angle of 90 degrees. You can release your pinched-up skin when you've finished your injection and removed the needle from your skin.

The pinch-up technique prevents you from injecting into muscle, but you may not need to use it if you use short needles or have a deep layer of subcutaneous fat.

■ **45-DEGREE TECHNIQUE** This involves inserting the needle directly into your skin (without pinching up beforehand) at an angle of 45 degrees. This angle helps you avoid injecting too deeply and reaching the muscle beneath your subcutaneous fat layer if you are using 12.7mm needles.

Insulin and equipment care

The correct way to care for your unopened supply of insulin (whether in bottle, cartridge, or disposable device form) is to store it in a refrigerator at a temperature of 2–8°C (36–46°F) and to discard any insulin that has reached its expiration date (this should appear on the bottle or cartridge, or on the packet of disposable devices). Insulin that is frozen, exposed to high temperatures or direct sunlight, or out of date does not work effectively and should be thrown away.

The insulin that you are using currently (whether in a bottle, or a reusable or disposable device) can be safely kept unrefrigerated at room temperature (up to 25°C/77°F) for one month. The advantage is that, if you're not in a hot climate, you can carry your insulin around with you without needing to keep it cool. You don't need to inject cold insulin that has come right from the refrigerator, which can be uncomfortable. If you are in a hot climate, you can keep insulin cool by storing it in a cool bag or bottle (see p.124).

HOW TO USE A SYRINGE

Check the appearance and expiration date of your insulin before you inject yourself. Discard insulin that is out of date or that looks different from usual. Make sure that the top of the insulin bottle is clean and use a new syringe each time you inject. This person is using the pinch-up technique (see opposite).

1 For cloudy insulin, invert the bottle so it is uniformly cloudy. Uncap the needle, and draw air into the syringe to match the insulin required. Insert the needle into the bottle and inject the air into the bottle.

2 Turn the bottle upside down and check that the tip of the needle is in the insulin. Then, pull the plunger back to draw up insulin into the syringe. When you have drawn up the correct dose of insulin, withdraw the needle from the insulin bottle.

3 Remove any air bubbles by holding the syringe with the needle upward and flicking the bubbles to the needle end before gently pressing on the plunger to push them out. Check that you still have the correct dose of insulin in the syringe.

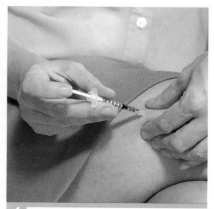

4 Pinch up a fold of skin at your chosen injection site (in this case the thigh) and insert the needle at a 90-degree angle to your body. Press the plunger to deliver the insulin. After injecting, remove the syringe and dispose of it safely (see p.100).

Two recent
advances that
may offer a
realistic way
of improving
diabetes control
and delivering
insulin are
delivering insulin
by inhaler and
transplanting
islet cells into
the pancreas.

Disposing of equipment safely

Syringes with integral needles and attachable needles for insulin devices are designed to be used once only. Reused needles can bend or become blunt, especially if they are very short or fine, and this can make injections uncomfortable. Also, with syringes, the dose markings may wear off with frequent reuse.

When you have finished with a device or syringe and needle, it's important to dispose of it safely to prevent injuries to yourself or others. You can do this by putting needles, syringes, and lancets into a puncture-proof heavy plastic or metal container with a tight-fitting lid, known as a sharps container. Alternatively, you can use a needle-clipping device; after you have clipped the needle from the syringe or device, it is retained in an inaccessible, puncture-proof compartment. A needle-clipping device has the advantage of being small and portable and enables you to use a new needle for each injection when you are out.

Safe disposal of sharps is a responsibility that should be taken seriously by people with diabetes. If you have diabetes, you should ask your healthcare professional about the best methods for storage and disposal of sharps. You should also check with your local health department regarding the disposal of your sharps containers—some municipalities have specific laws about the disposal of medical waste.

Recent advances in treatment

From time to time, media headlines highlight research that claims to successfully treat or cure diabetes. This may include transplanting of non-insulin-producing cells, which can be altered to enable them to produce insulin, or devices that can automatically deliver the right amount of insulin in response to your changing blood glucose level. Such research is usually in the very early stages, however, and may never develop fully to become a realistic treatment for most people with diabetes. Your health professional will help you identify which treatments are likely to be available to you and also which are likely to be of benefit to you.

Two recent advances in treatment that may offer a realistic way of improving diabetes control and delivering insulin are delivering insulin via inhaler and transplanting islet cells into the pancreas.

Inhaled insulin

Many people who have asthma take their treatment by inhaler. Now the same idea is being applied to insulin. Several insulin manufacturers have designed electronic inhalers that deliver insulin to the lungs as a powder or fine stream of liquid. The insulin comes in a sachet or strip containing a set dose—you insert as many of these as you need into the inhaler. People with type 1 and type 2 diabetes could use inhaled insulin but, because the insulin is of the fast-acting type (see p.85), people with type 1 diabetes (and some people with type 2) still need an injection of long-acting insulin.

Insulin inhalers are large electronic devices because they need to contain equipment that monitors the amount of insulin entering your lungs. As with injected insulin, the amount of insulin you inhale is critical: too much and you may experience hypoglycemia, too little and you risk hyperglycemia.

Trials in the US, Canada, and Europe suggest that inhalation could be an effective way of taking insulin, although more research is necessary to find out the effect of insulin on the lungs and how well inhaled insulin can control your blood glucose.

Islet cell transplant

If you have type 1 diabetes, the insulin-producing beta cells, found in the islet cells in your pancreas, have been destroyed. Efforts have been made to overcome this problem by transplanting islet cells or even the entire pancreas.

However, transplanting a whole pancreas is a difficult operation and can often be unsuccessful. Islet cell transplants offer a greater chance of success. Islet cells are injected into a vein that leads to the liver, which is a simple procedure that does not require a general anesthetic. The cells settle in the liver and begin to produce insulin. Most people have been found to need at least two or three transplants of islet cells before they can control their blood glucose level without insulin injections. In some cases, the body's immune system may treat transplanted cells as though they are foreign invaders and attack them. Because of this, islet cells need to be specially treated before they are transplanted. Also, ongoing development of anti-rejection treatment has increased the chances of the cells being accepted by the person's body.

Only a small number of people have so far had islet cell transplants using this technique, and although the success of islet cell transplant has encouraged many health care sites to perform this procedure, it is still considered experimental in nature.

It will be some time before the majority of people living with diabetes can reap the benefits of the research that is taking place, and the procedure itself still has to undergo further lengthy trials.

The possible side effects of the autoimmune drugs that are used to prevent the transplanted cells being rejected by the body also require close monitoring.

My experience

"The fact that some people have had islet cell transplants gives me great hope. Even if it's not for me, it might help the kids who are being diagnosed today." JOE

COMMENT Islet cell transplants and complete pancreas transplants offer hope that diabetes may be cured in the future, even though it will be many years until treatments like this are available to most people with diabetes.

Myth OR TRUTH?

MYTH
An islet cell transplant cures diabetes.

TRUTH
People who have had an islet cell transplant are often able to stop injecting insulin since they start producing enough insulin to control their blood glucose level. It is too early to say whether they will be free of injections on a permanent basis.

Hypoglycemia

If you take insulin or insulin-stimulating pills for your diabetes, your blood glucose level may sometimes fall too low—this is known as hypoglycemia. Being aware of the factors that trigger hypoglycemia can help you prevent it from happening. If you do have a hypoglycemic reaction, recognizing the symptoms as soon as possible enables you to treat yourself quickly and easily. If the reaction becomes more severe, you may need other people to help you treat it.

If you do have a hypoglycemic reaction, identify the cause so that you can take steps to prevent the same situation from occurring again.

What is hypoglycemia?

Hypoglycemia is the term used to describe a blood glucose level that is too low. In practical terms, this means any level below 4 millimoles per liter, although the level at which the symptoms of hypoglycemia occur can vary from person to person. These low blood levels occur when there is more insulin in your body than you need at the time.

If you take insulin, you are sure to experience hypoglycemia occasionally. You are also at risk for hypoglycemia if you take insulin-stimulating pills such as sulfonylureas, but not other pills for diabetes, such as metformin, thiazolidinediones, or alpha-glucosidase inhibitors, on their own (see pp.76–81).

It is important to try to prevent hypoglycemia or treat it promptly because a very low blood glucose level can make you feel ill, keep you from thinking clearly, and make your blood glucose level erratic. If it is severe, you may lose consciousness.

Treatment for a hypoglycemic episode consists of eating or drinking glucose, then eating a carbohydrate-containing snack or meal. If you lose consciousness, you will need an injection of glucagon or glucose (see p.109) to raise your blood glucose level. Even after you have treated, or been treated for, hypoglycemia and your blood glucose level is back within the normal range, you may need some time to recover.

Causes and prevention

A hypoglycemic reaction happens when you have too much insulin in your body, perhaps because your insulin or pill dose doesn't match your food intake or your level of activity. It can also happen if

FITTING IN FOOD
A busy lifestyle can sometimes make it difficult to fit regular meals into your day. Missing or delaying eating, however, puts you at risk of hypoglycemia, so you need to be aware of when to eat, and ensure that you do so, in order to prevent or treat a hypoglycemic reaction.

you have taken an incorrect dose. If you do have a hypoglycemic reaction, identify the cause so that you can take steps to prevent the same situation from occurring again.

■ **INSULIN AND PILL DOSE** If you regularly have the symptoms of hypoglycemia, you may need a lower dose of insulin or insulin-stimulating pills. Dose reductions are commonly needed if you lose weight, you are eating less than usual, you become more physically active, or you have successfully taken a higher dose of insulin to control a high blood glucose level. If you inject yourself with insulin or take insulin-stimulating pills several times a day, it's important to identify which injection or pill is responsible for a hypoglycemic reaction, and then adjust that dose. For example, if your blood glucose level falls before lunch on a few consecutive days, you need to reduce your morning dose of insulin or insulin-stimulating pills.

■ **FOOD INTAKE** Injected insulin and insulin-stimulating pills work over a number of hours to control your blood glucose level, and you need to eat during this time to prevent your blood glucose level from falling too low. If you inject insulin, you need to know whether it has a peak action and, if so, when this is, so that you can balance it with a carbohydrate snack. If you don't balance your insulin dose with carbohydrate-containing food at the right time, you risk having a hypoglycemic reaction. Eating later or less than usual, missing a snack, or eating a different type of food, without knowing how much carbohydrate it contains, can increase your risk of having hypoglycemia. If you are unsure about the timing of meals and snacks for your particular insulin regimen, ask your health professional.

■ **ALCOHOL** Although, initially, alcohol causes your blood glucose level to

---

Practical tips

PREVENTING & TREATING HYPOGLYCEMIA

● Check your blood glucose level several hours after strenuous activity.

● If you find it helpful, ask friends, family, or colleagues to remind you to test your blood glucose or to eat snacks at the right times.

● Keep glucose and carbohydrate-containing snacks handy at home, at work, in your car, and in your pocket or handbag.

● If you suspect your blood glucose level is falling, do a blood test to check.

My experience

"Like many people who have diabetes, I'm frightened of developing complications and I try to reduce my risk by tightly controlling my blood glucose level. I quickly realized, however, that having hypoglycemia was the downside of such tight control." STUART

COMMENT Although hypoglycemia is more likely when your diabetes is well controlled, it isn't inevitable. One solution is to change to a different type of insulin or pill. Your health professional will advise you.

rise, over a period of hours it causes your blood glucose level to fall. This puts you at risk of a hypoglycemic episode if you take insulin or insulin-stimulating pills. Such episodes are particularly dangerous when you have been drinking because alcohol impairs the corrective mechanism that normally occurs during a hypoglycemic reaction, in which the liver's store of glycogen is converted back to glucose and released into the bloodstream. In some situations, hypoglycemia as a result of alcohol consumption can be life-threatening.

You can prevent this by never drinking on an empty stomach. If you have more than 2 drinks of alcohol, eat extra carbohydrate-containing food to compensate. This extra food could be potato chips, a sandwich, or a take-out meal.

■ **PHYSICAL ACTIVITY** Any sort of physical activity, whether housework, shopping, swimming, or tennis, requires energy. Your body's primary source of energy is glucose and the more active you are, the more glucose you burn and the more your blood glucose level falls. You can prevent a hypoglycemic reaction in this situation by reducing the dose of your insulin or insulin-stimulating pills before physical activity or by eating extra food before, during, or after activity. Long-lasting or strenuous activity requires more careful planning (see pp.58–59).

Staying active helps all your body systems work more efficiently and is important for your long-term health. With careful preparation you can prevent your blood glucose level from falling (see pp.56–58).

■ **STRESS** Stress usually makes your blood glucose level rise because the stress hormones epinephrine (adrenaline) and cortisol not only oppose the action of insulin, but also cause glycogen in your liver to be converted into glucose and released into your bloodstream. However, stress can also cause your blood glucose level to fall because your body may use extra energy when you are stressed or you may not eat regularly. Try to establish the effect of stress on your blood glucose level. If you know that it lowers your blood glucose level, you can deal with stressful situations by eating extra food or reducing the dose of your insulin or insulin-stimulating pills.

■ **HEAT** Exposure to heat causes your blood to circulate more quickly, and therefore insulin and insulin-stimulating pills work faster than usual. This in turn causes your blood glucose level to fall. You may find that you are prone to low blood glucose levels in hot weather. Checking your blood glucose before taking a hot bath, sauna, or using a sunbed will help you determine whether you are close to a hypoglycemic episode and whether you need extra food to avoid this. You may need to reduce your dose of insulin or insulin-stimulating pills or eat extra food before or after these activities.

Symptoms

The symptoms of hypoglycemia fall into two categories: early warning symptoms, when your blood glucose level starts to drop, and later symptoms, when it is so low that your brain is not receiving sufficient glucose. The symptoms are more pronounced for some people than for others. If you can't detect and treat your own symptoms, you may need to rely on people around you for help.

Early warning symptoms

You may have any of the following symptoms when your blood glucose level starts to fall:
- Sweating
- Trembling
- Feeling anxious
- Turning pale
- Palpitations
- Feeling hungry

You may not have all or even any of these symptoms; it's also possible to experience these symptoms in response to any drop in blood glucose—for example, a drop from 15 millimoles per liter to

10 millimoles per liter. Testing your blood glucose level will give you the information you need to decide whether any action is necessary. Bear in mind, though, that a blood glucose test result does not reveal how quickly your blood glucose level is changing—if you have symptoms and your test result is 4 millimoles per liter, treat yourself for hypoglycemia immediately rather than waiting for it to drop further.

Later symptoms

As your blood glucose level falls below 3 millimoles per liter, your brain is no longer receiving a sufficient amount of glucose. Although you may know that you are having a hypoglycemic reaction, you may not be able to think clearly enough to treat yourself. You may experience one or more of the following symptoms:
- Difficulty concentrating
- Feeling disoriented
- Acting out of character
- Being aggressive
- Being uncooperative
- Blurred vision
- Headache

If you are too confused to treat yourself, you need the help of people around you. This can be problematic, since you may be uncooperative and reluctant to accept help. However, relatives, friends, and colleagues can become skilled at both recognizing the signs of a hypoglycemic episode and urging you to accept treatment. If you don't treat or receive treatment for your hypoglycemia and your

Myth or TRUTH?

MYTH
If hypoglycemic episodes occur during the night and you don't wake up, you can die.

TRUTH
Hypoglycemic symptoms usually wake you up, but even if they don't, glycogen will be converted to glucose in your liver and released into your bloodstream, correcting your blood glucose level. Excess insulin also wears off naturally in time. Hypoglycemia can be life-threatening if you have been drinking large amounts of alcohol on an empty stomach because alcohol impairs this corrective mechanism.

blood glucose level continues to fall, you may lose consciousness. Getting to this stage normally takes quite a while after early warning symptoms start—up to 2 hours—but it may happen within 10 to 15 minutes of having the later symptoms.

Reduced awareness of symptoms

If you have a series of frequent hypoglycemic episodes—for example, three or four times over a two-week period —your body gets used to the low blood glucose level and is slower at giving you early warning symptoms. By the time you realize what is happening, your blood glucose level may have fallen below 3 millimoles per liter. At this point you are likely to find it difficult to treat yourself.

If you have had diabetes for years and have often had hypoglycemic reactions, you may not get any early warning symptoms at all. Your only symptoms of hypoglycemia may be confusion and disorientation, by which point it could be too late to treat the attack yourself; you may

> If you have had diabetes for years and have often had hypoglycemic episodes, your body may not give you any early warning symptoms at all.

lose consciousness if you don't receive help. If you experience frequent hypoglycemic episodes and reduced awareness of symptoms, your health professional may suggest that you temporarily relax your diabetes control and allow your blood glucose level to rise above the ideal range of 4–7 millimoles per liter—to 10 millimoles or more per liter, for example. This provides a respite from hypoglycemia and can also help restore your awareness of symptoms.

Treatment

There are two stages to treating hypoglycemia: first, eat or drink glucose as soon as possible, and then, eat a more substantial carbohydrate-containing food to prevent your blood glucose level from falling again. If you lose consciousness, you will need help from someone else.

Initial treatment

As soon as you realize that you are hypoglycemic, you need to eat or drink something that is high in glucose—any of the following will start to raise your blood glucose level quickly (within 10–15 minutes):

- 15g of glucose in the form of glucose tablets.
- 15mL (3 teaspoons) or 3 packets of table sugar dissolved in water.
- 175mL (¾ cup) of juice or regular soft drink.
- 3 Life Savers® (1 = 2.5g of carbohydrate).
- 15mL (1 tablespoon) of honey.

My experience

"I've learned not to eat too much when I have a low blood glucose level—15–20 grams of carbohydrate is enough. This keeps my blood glucose from getting too high afterward." LOUISE

COMMENT It takes experience to know how much carbohydrate you need for the secondary treatment of a hypoglycemic reaction. If you eat too much, you may get hyperglycemia. Checking your blood glucose level when you feel better will tell you whether you have taken enough.

Q If I pass out from hypoglycemia in a public place and I'm not with my family or friends, how will anyone know what's wrong with me?

A Ambulance crew or hospital staff would automatically test your blood glucose level to determine whether hypoglycemia is the cause of your unconsciousness. If you take insulin or insulin-stimulating pills, always carry identification giving details of your diabetes and treatment, such as an identification card or a special bracelet, to make sure that you are treated accurately and as quickly as possible.

If you take insulin or insulin-stimulating pills, you should carry an emergency supply of glucose with you at all times. You may find a particular form and amount of glucose that suits you better, but remember that some glucose-rich food and drinks, such as chocolate or milky drinks that contain sugar, also contain fat, which slows their absorption into your bloodstream.

Secondary treatment

After taking glucose, you will need to eat something more substantial that contains carbohydrate and a protein source, particularly if your next meal is more than an hour away.

The exact amount of food you need depends on the circumstances of your hypoglycemic reaction. This carbohydrate-containing food prevents your blood glucose level from falling again after your body has used up the glucose taken previously. If a hypoglycemic episode occurs just before a meal, take the initial treatment and let the meal act as the secondary treatment. The most important thing is to detect and treat hypoglycemia promptly, taking steps to produce the fastest rise in blood glucose to a safe level.

If you lose consciousness

If you are unconscious or losing consciousness, it is dangerous to try to eat or drink anything because you won't be able to swallow properly and you may choke. Instead, you need an injection of either glucagon or glucose. Glucagon raises your blood glucose level by causing glycogen in your liver to be quickly converted into glucose and released into your bloodstream. An injection of glucagon will usually have an effect within 10 minutes. If you are

SECONDARY TREATMENT
Family and friends who know how to deal with hypoglycemia will be able to help you when you need it, such as by giving you additional carbohydrate.

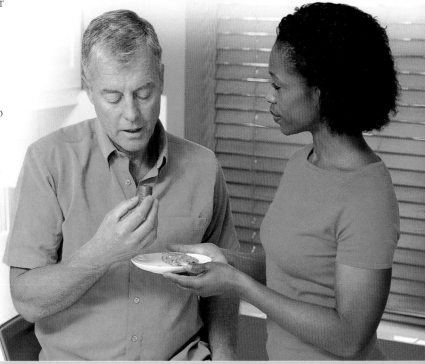

at risk of losing consciousness during a hypoglycemic attack, your health professional can prescribe glucagon. A friend can be shown how to test your blood glucose and how to inject glucagon (see box, opposite). A glucose injection under your skin or into a vein in your arm can be given by ambulance crew or hospital staff, to help you regain consciousness within 5–10 minutes. Whether you receive a glucagon or glucose injection, you need a carbohydrate snack or meal, since the glucose in your bloodstream is used up quickly.

Getting help

If you take insulin or insulin-stimulating pills, it's important to inform your family and friends about early warning symptoms, later symptoms, and the treatment of hypoglycemia. This way, if you need help during an episode, people know how to recognize it and what action to take. Others you may want to inform about the possibility of hypoglycemia are colleagues and people with whom you are drinking alcohol (alcohol increases the risk of hypoglycemia, see pp.103–104).

The recovery period

Even if you don't receive treatment for hypoglycemia, your body eventually takes corrective action to raise the level of glucose in your blood. The glycogen in your liver is converted into glucose and released into your bloodstream to raise your blood glucose level. The effect of your insulin or insulin-stimulating pills also wears off. This causes your blood glucose level to rise. So, although it is not ideal, even if you lose consciousness and there is no one around to help you, you will regain consciousness naturally within an hour or two. There are exceptions to this, however: if you have a very large amount of insulin and/or alcohol in your bloodstream, your hypoglycemic attack will last much longer and will be more severe.

During the recovery period, your blood glucose level may become too high as a result of the extra glucose that you have produced and consumed. This reaction is known as "rebound hyperglycemia" and it can

---

TREATING HYPOGLYCEMIA: A CONSCIOUS PERSON

A relative, friend, or colleague who takes insulin or insulin-stimulating pills may have an occasional hypoglycemic episode. If the person is confused and unable to treat himself, you may need to treat him.

1 If a person is showing early symptoms of hypoglycemia (see p.105), get him to test his blood glucose before treating him. If he is showing later symptoms of hypoglycemia (see p.105), give him 3 glucose pills or a sugar drink.

2 If he starts to feel better quickly, give him a carbohydrate snack, such as crackers and cheese. Don't give any food or drink if you suspect he is losing consciousness; follow the procedure for dealing with someone unconscious (see box opposite).

TREATING HYPOGLYCEMIA: AN UNCONSCIOUS PERSON

If hypoglycemia is untreated and blood glucose continues to fall, the person may lose consciousness. In this situation, you need to give a glucagon injection. Glucagon kits can be prescribed and should be stored in a refrigerator.

1 Put the person on his side, placing his arm and leg at right angles to his body. Tilt his head back to keep his airway clear.

2 If you have access to a glucagon injection kit, remove the seal on the glucagon bottle. Uncap the needle, put it into the bottle, and inject the water from the syringe into the bottle.

3 Rotate the bottle until all the glucagon powder has dissolved. Turn it upside down and check that the needle tip is in the solution. Pull the plunger to withdraw all the solution (it should fill the syringe to the 1mL mark).

4 Insert the needle at a right angle into the person's thigh, buttock, or arm, and depress the plunger to inject. Withdraw the needle, press a tissue or swab on the injection site, and keep him in the recovery position until he is conscious.

> During the recovery period, your blood glucose level may become too high as a result of the extra glucose that you have produced and consumed.

happen shortly after a hypoglycemic reaction or during the next 24 hours.

If you take fast-acting insulin, you can use a small dose to correct rebound hyperglycemia. However, increasing your dose of other types of insulin may encourage further attacks because other insulins have a longer action. Instead, figure out the cause of the hypoglycemia and take steps to prevent it from happening again (see pp.102–105).

Even after you have treated a hypoglycemic episode and your blood glucose level is above 4 millimoles per liter, it may take several hours for you to recover completely. In particular, you may feel ill and find it difficult to concentrate.

Hyperglycemia

When you have diabetes, your body cells cannot take in glucose from your bloodstream. As a result, the level of glucose in your blood remains high, a condition known as hyperglycemia. Your diabetes treatment is aimed at reducing hyperglycemia and preventing your blood glucose from becoming too high (more than 7 millimoles per liter) on a regular basis. This helps protect against short- and long-term complications. You can take action to treat hyperglycemia according to its cause.

What is hyperglycemia?

Hyperglycemia is the term used to describe an elevated blood glucose level (above 7 millimoles per liter). It is the main effect of untreated diabetes and, therefore, it may have been the symptoms of hyperglycemia that led you to seek help when you were first diagnosed with diabetes.

Hyperglycemia can not only make you feel unwell in the short-term, but also, if it happens frequently, it increases your risk of the long-term

The most obvious causes of hyperglycemia are either an increase in the amount of food you eat or a decrease in your level of activity.

Q Can losing weight help me to prevent hyperglycemia?

A If you have a lot of body fat, your body needs a greater amount of insulin to control your blood glucose, so hyperglycemia is more likely. If your BMI is in the recommended range (see p.46), your body is able to use insulin more efficiently than if you are overweight.

complications of diabetes. This is why a blood glucose level of 4–7 millimoles per liter is usually recommended for good diabetes control.

Although the main goal of diabetes treatment is to prevent hyperglycemia, an occasional raised blood glucose level (7–10 millimoles per liter) is to be expected when you have diabetes. Even when you control your blood glucose level most of the time, there are occasions when stress, illness, or not getting the right dose of insulin or pills, for example, can raise your blood glucose level.

Hyperglycemia can affect anyone with diabetes, whether you use insulin or pills, or manage your diabetes with a healthy diet and physical activity.

Causes and prevention

A key aspect of diabetes control is understanding what makes your blood glucose level rise and taking

MONITORING DURING ILLNESS
When you are ill, your blood glucose level rises and can quickly get out of control. This is why it's very important to test your blood glucose level frequently and adjust your diabetes treatment accordingly.

action to keep this from happening. Regularly checking your blood glucose level to see if it is within the target range of 4–7 millimoles per liter can give you the information you need to prevent hyperglycemia.

If you have a raised blood glucose level on a number of occasions—for example, if your test results are often 8–9 millimoles per liter—it's time to act quickly. Don't wait until you experience symptoms, because by this time your blood glucose level is likely to be 10 millimoles per liter or above.

■ **FOOD INTAKE/PHYSICAL ACTIVITY**
The most obvious causes of hyperglycemia are either an increase in the amount of food you eat (resulting in extra glucose entering your bloodstream) or a decrease in your level of activity (resulting in decreased use of glucose by your body cells). Eating certain types of food—those that are high in sugar,

for example—can also lead to an elevated blood glucose level. Ways of preventing hyperglycemia include following healthy eating guidelines (see pp.30–43) and staying active (see pp.52–59).

■ **ILLNESS** When you are ill, glycogen in your liver is converted to glucose and released into your bloodstream. Increased amounts of the stress hormones cortisol and epinephrine (adrenaline) are also produced. These hormones prevent your insulin from working efficiently.

Both these processes cause your blood glucose level to rise. Frequent blood glucose monitoring is very important when you are ill because it enables you to react quickly and make the appropriate adjustments to your diabetes treatment.

■ **STRESS/HORMONAL CHANGES** Stress hormones can oppose the action of insulin in your body so that your blood glucose level rises as

Practical tips

PREVENTING HYPERGLYCEMIA

● Try to avoid overeating or, if you know you are going to eat more than usual, adjust your insulin or pills (or increase your level of activity).

● Be aware of the effect of stress and other hormonal changes on your blood glucose level so that you can predict when you need to adjust your treatment.

● Don't stop taking your insulin/pills when you are sick (especially if you have a vomiting illness) and monitor your blood glucose level frequently.

● Take your insulin or pills every day and adjust the dose when necessary.

a result. Also, when you are stressed you may overeat or eat less healthy types of food. This can cause your blood glucose to rise. If you are a woman, you may find that your blood glucose level rises at certain stages of your menstrual cycle (particularly just before periods). Hormonal changes during menopause can also result in hyperglycemia.

Some hormonal conditions (see p.17), such as Cushing disease and acromegaly, are also associated with hyperglycemia, because they affect the efficiency of insulin. If you find that hormonal changes raise your blood glucose level, increase your frequency of blood glucose monitoring at the appropriate time— before your menstrual period, for example—and take action quickly.

■ **INSULIN/DIABETES PILLS** If you haven't been able to take your insulin or pills for any reason, your blood glucose level rises. Sometimes, you may have hyperglycemia even though you have taken your insulin or pills correctly; this suggests that you may need a different dose or type of insulin or pill. If you have type 2 diabetes that you manage with a healthy diet and physical activity and your blood

> **If you are a woman, you may find that your blood glucose level rises at certain stages of your menstrual cycle.**

glucose level is frequently elevated, you may need to start taking pills; talk to your health professional.

Symptoms

The symptoms of hyperglycemia are the same as those you may have had when your diabetes was first diagnosed (see pp.18–19). Possible symptoms include:

- Frequent urination
- Dry mouth, excessive thirst
- Lack of energy
- Weight loss
- Blurred vision
- Yeast and cystitis.

Hyperglycemia may also be symptomless, especially if you have type 2 diabetes or your body is used to an elevated blood glucose level.

Treatment

You need to tailor your treatment of hyperglycemia to its cause. This could mean decreasing your food intake, increasing your level of physical activity and/or increasing your insulin or pill dosage (for information about adjusting your insulin dose, see pp.90–95). If you have type 2 diabetes that you manage by eating a healthy diet and physical activity, you may need to start taking pills if your blood glucose level is consistently above 7 millimoles per liter. If you are ill, prompt treatment for your illness will limit the effect of hyperglycemia (see pp.130–133). Whatever action you take to treat

---

My experience

"I know my blood glucose rises when I'm ill, even if I eat less, so I check my blood glucose 7–8 times a day and adjust my insulin accordingly." SOPHIE

COMMENT If you experience hyperglycemia when you are ill, it is important to adjust your treatment promptly when your blood glucose level is high, to prevent it from becoming an emergency situation.

hyperglycemia, test your blood glucose level frequently to check that it is returning to normal. If your blood glucose level falls as a result of increasing your dose of insulin or insulin-stimulating pills, you may need to reduce the dosage once your blood glucose level is back in the recommended range.

If you cannot establish the cause of your hyperglycemia, or you are unsure how to treat it, talk to your health professional. Hyperglycemia should always be treated promptly to avoid both short- and long-term complications.

Risks

An occasional, brief spell of hyperglycemia may be uncomfortable, but is not likely to be harmful. However, a consistently high or rising blood glucose level can cause short- and long-term complications.

Short-term risks

If hyperglycemia is untreated and your blood glucose level continues to rise (above 20 millimoles per liter), you may develop diabetic ketoacidosis if you have type 1 diabetes, or nonketotic hyperosmolar state if you have type 2 diabetes.

■ **DIABETIC KETOACIDOSIS (DKA)** If there is no insulin in your body, your body cells are unable to take in glucose from your bloodstream. This means that your body is deprived of its primary source of energy and is forced to break down fat as an alternative energy source. During fat breakdown, toxic by-products that are known as ketones are produced. An excessive amount of ketones in the body can make your blood highly acidic and cause symptoms such as nausea, vomiting, abdominal pain, and fruity-smelling breath (as a result of your body trying to expel ketones through your lungs). Untreated DKA can lead to coma and may occasionally be fatal. DKA is a medical emergency and needs to be treated in the hospital. Treatment consists of an insulin infusion via a vein (see pp.134–135), intravenous fluids, potassium, and substances to correct the acidity of your blood.

■ **NONKETOTIC HYPEROSMOLAR STATE** If you have type 2 diabetes, you are unlikely to develop DKA. This is because you still produce insulin, and your body has access to some glucose as an energy source and is not entirely dependent on fat as an alternative. However, severe hyperglycemia can lead to excessive dehydration and occasionally coma, which is known as a nonketotic hyperosmolar state. This is also very serious and needs to be treated in the hospital.

Long-term risks

If your blood glucose level is elevated over an extended period of months and years, you have a greater risk of developing the long-term complications of diabetes. These include eye, kidney, and heart disease, and damage to the nervous system (see pp.186–215).

Myth OR TRUTH?

MYTH
If I feel well, it means that I don't have a high blood glucose level.

TRUTH
If your blood glucose level has been higher than normal, for example 10–15 millimoles per liter, for more than a few days, you may not feel ill or have symptoms. Your body may have become accustomed to a higher-than-normal blood glucose level and adjusted. If this happens, you don't have symptoms until your blood glucose level is even higher. This is why you should always rely on blood glucose monitoring rather than symptoms to detect hyperglycemia.

Living with diabetes

In most cases, diabetes is a lifelong condition, so it's essential to learn how to incorporate diabetes care into your daily life. Diabetes affects many aspects of your day-to-day life—from working to driving, going on vacation to having sex. In all of these instances, being informed and planning ahead will help you anticipate and prevent problems.

Looking after yourself when you have diabetes includes taking care of your feet daily, and making sure that you take extra care of your diabetes when you are ill. Going into a hospital may also mean that you need a change in your diabetes management.

If you are a woman with diabetes, there are times when you need to be extra careful about monitoring your blood glucose level and tailoring your treatment to the results. Conception and pregnancy are times when tight control of your diabetes is essential. Gestational diabetes (diabetes that occurs during pregnancy) also needs careful treatment.

Living with diabetes involves regular contact with health professionals who provide help and support. It's useful to plan ahead before your appointments, so that you can get the most from your health care.

Day-to-day life

Looking after your diabetes every single day can require an effort of will, and learning how to motivate yourself to keep going is very important. Diabetes might affect you in your line of work, when driving a vehicle, and when traveling, and knowing how to deal with different situations will make it far less likely that diabetes will restrict you. Diabetes also affects the people you are close to, your relationships, and specific aspects of women's health and pregnancy.

Staying motivated

Diabetes is very different from a short-term illness, for which you might need, for example, a course of antibiotics, a short stay in a hospital, or even an operation. In such circumstances, you expect the treatment to cure your illness and return you to full health, which helps motivate you to do whatever is necessary to recover. Once you have diabetes, unless it is gestational diabetes, you have it for life. Any care or treatment you receive is designed not to cure you but to prevent short-term problems, such as uncomfortable symptoms of hyperglycemia, and the long-term complications of diabetes that could develop over years to come. While you can do much to protect yourself against complications, there is no guarantee that you won't develop problems at some point in your life. All this means that caring for your diabetes day after day requires lots of motivation. Feelings of despondency about the amount of effort you have to put in are entirely normal. Developing coping strategies to see you through the difficult times can help you keep going.

Coping in the long term

There are a number of obstacles, perceived or real, that might get in the way of your diabetes care, such as:
● Being unable to identify when your blood glucose level is creeping up, because you still feel well.
● Not finding time to monitor your blood glucose level.

My experience

"Sometimes I feel like I'm in a straitjacket— I get sick and tired of caring for my diabetes and there are never any vacations." JOE

COMMENT You may feel that looking after your diabetes is a burden. If you feel trapped, taking time to identify your specific concerns and devising a plan of action to overcome obstacles can help refresh your motivation.

LIVING LIFE TO THE FULL
Having diabetes doesn't mean that you can't go out and enjoy yourself, although sometimes you will need to plan ahead or make some last-minute adjustments. Knowing about diabetes can help you work out a strategy for any situation you find yourself in.

• Forgetting to, or not being able to, take your medication when you are supposed to.

• Having to eat what everyone else eats, healthy or not.

• Fitting in with others; not wanting to upset them.

• Not wanting to be different.

• Becoming fed up with your day-to-day routine.

• Feeling as though nothing you do makes a difference to your blood glucose level.

One way of tackling such obstacles is to follow a four-step action plan to help you make positive changes. Start by identifying the obstacle, explore how it makes you feel, consider ways to solve it, and finally decide what you will do to overcome it.

■ **WHAT GETS IN THE WAY?** Write down all the times you find it difficult to look after your diabetes, and try to identify what exactly is getting in the way.

■ **HOW DOES IT MAKE YOU FEEL?** Consider how you feel about situations that prevent you from looking after your diabetes. If your feelings are negative, acknowledging this can be a very important step.

■ **WHAT ARE YOUR OPTIONS?** Think about what you could do to change things for the better. You might have some ideas about this already. Visualize what you would like to have happen and what options you have to bring this about.

■ **WHAT ARE YOU GOING TO DO?** Plan how you are going to bring about change. The more specific your plan, the more likely you are to achieve it. For example, if you want to lose weight, set yourself a target and a time scale and then break them down into smaller chunks to help you identify a weekly weight loss target. Then work out what changes you need to make on a daily basis to achieve this. If you want to remember

Write down all the times you find it difficult to look after your diabetes, and try to identify what exactly is getting in the way.

to take your pills more regularly, for example, the first step is to set a realistic goal of how many days a week you will take all your pills. The next step is to work out how you are going to achieve this on each of these days. To help you plan, ask yourself the following questions:

- What exactly are you going to do?
- When will you start?
- Do you need to do anything to prepare for it beforehand?
- What will get in the way of you achieving it?
- How can you reduce the chances of anything getting in the way?

Ask yourself if what you have planned is really possible. If not, set yourself smaller targets to ensure success. Monitor your progress to check that you are on target for success. If you are succeeding, you need to congratulate yourself. If you haven't quite succeeded, try not to get discourageed. Instead, review your options, identify one that is realistic and achievable, and set yourself a different goal and timeframe. If you are still struggling to achieve your goals, you could ask someone close to you to help, perhaps to monitor your progress or to talk through whatever it is that you find difficult. Changing your behavior takes time, so be prepared—and keep trying.

> **If you manage your diabetes with healthy eating and physical activity, there should be no restrictions on the type of work you do.**

Peer-Support Groups

It is not unusual to feel scared, shocked, overwhelmed, or even angry when you first hear that you have diabetes. A positive and realistic attitude toward your diabetes can help you to maintain good blood glucose levels. Blood glucose levels in your target range can help delay, or even prevent, diabetes complications.

Talk to others who have diabetes—ask your local Canadian Diabetes Association branch about joining a peer-support group or visiting an information session.

Peer-support groups give people who share a similar relationship to diabetes an opportunity to regularly share their experiences and support each other, thereby enabling them to successfully live with their disease.

Support and information

Peer-support groups help to:
- increase participants' knowledge in areas of diabetes management.
- create a greater comfort level in dealing with the emotional aspects of diabetes.
- make healthy life style changes.
- enlarge support networks.
- increase awareness of the Canadian Diabetes Association and other

---

My experience

"My husband really understands my concerns and the issues that frighten me. He sits down and talks to me about how we can deal with things together." SOPHIE

COMMENT Having the support of someone close to you can help you cope more easily when times are difficult. You could ask your partner to monitor your progress if you are trying to make changes, or simply to talk through any aspects of your diabetes care that are worrying you.

Q Is there anything I can do if I believe that I am being turned down for a job simply because I have diabetes?

A If you think that you are being denied a job because you have diabetes, your potential employer should be able to provide concrete reasons why the position would not be suitable for you. If you believe that their reasons are discriminatory, you can contact the Canadian Diabetes Association to discuss your situation. The organization may provide support if you decide to pursue your case. There have been several successful court cases in which people with diabetes have proved that they can do their jobs just as well as people without diabetes.

diabetes services that are available in the area.

Peer-Support Groups are managed by the volunteer peer-facilitator(s). The participants determine the format, direction, and topics raised in the group. The groups meet regularly (often monthly) and participants are expected to commit to the life of the group (often from fall to spring).

Work

There are very few jobs that you cannot do if you have diabetes. If you manage your diabetes with healthy eating and physical activity, there should be no restrictions on the type of work that you do. By keeping your diabetes well controlled, you can make sure that it does not affect your performance at work. It may even have a positive influence on colleagues as they see

that you can manage both your job and your diabetes without any problems.

Applying for jobs

When applying for a job, you are not required to inform your potential employers that you have diabetes—they cannot legally ask you about your health, or demand that you have a physical exam before they offer you the job.

You may feel reluctant to volunteer information about your condition, especially if you think you are less likely to be offered the job as a result, or you think your prospective employer might be concerned about the company's health insurance premiums being increased. If you are unsure, ask your health professional or contact the Canadian Diabetes Association for advice. However, once you are hired, telling your employer about your diabetes may enable you to eat when you need to at work without causing any difficulty, and to have time off if you need it for medical reasons. You should also tell your employer that you have diabetes if you take insulin or insulin-stimulating pills and you are responsible for other people's safety.

ATTENDING INTERVIEWS
Potential employers are unlikely to discriminate against you when you have diabetes, especially if you talk to them openly about how diabetes affects you and what can be expected of you.

Some potential employers may have justifiable concerns about your safety when carrying out certain tasks, such as driving, operating heavy machinery, or working at heights. In these circumstances you could be in danger if your medication puts you at risk of a low blood sugar reaction and you had one with very little warning. However, if you can demonstrate that your blood glucose is well controlled, through self-monitoring results and medical reports if necessary, even these jobs should be accessible to you.

Continuing in your existing job

If you discover that you have diabetes while already working in a restricted field of employment, you will not necessarily be dismissed.

Whether an employer will allow you to continue in your position will depend on the type of work you do, the extent to which diabetes affects it, and on the risk that your condition poses to yourself and others.

Blood glucose control

However busy your job, caring for your diabetes is important if you are to perform well; a high blood glucose level could affect your ability to perform by making you feel ill and a low level could lead to hypoglycemia.

Whether you have a regular schedule or one that changes from one day to the next, your diabetes

should not hold you back, provided that you can devise a routine to suit your diabetes and fit into your working day.

If the job that you do is quite unpredictable or involves a considerable amount of physical activity, you may need to check your blood glucose level three to four times during the working day. You may also need to find time for snacks or extra food at mealtimes. If you need to take insulin or insulin-stimulating pills at mealtimes, it's a good idea to keep a supply at work, along with some emergency low blood sugar remedies, such as glucose pills or drinks.

If you ever have hypoglycemic reactions without warning, then your colleagues should be told what they can do to help (see pp.106–109) if this occurs. Tell them what supplies you have for treating low blood sugar and where you keep them, and explain what colleagues might need to do if you are unable to deal with the attack yourself.

If your colleagues are concerned about your hypoglycemic episodes and their effect on your ability to do your job, your health professional should be able to work with you and your employer to find a way of dealing with your diabetes that enables you to do your job effectively and stay well. You could discuss a change of insulin or pill dose or type that would suit your work pattern better, or learn to recognize low blood sugar early.

Practical tips

COPING WITH SHIFT WORK

- Monitor your blood glucose to find out what effect working shifts has on your diabetes, so that you can adjust your pills or insulin accordingly.
- Remember that insulin and pills need to be taken in relation to your food intake as opposed to the time of day.
- If break times or the type of work you do are subject to change at short notice, make sure you always have glucose and carbohydrate snacks with you if you take insulin or insulin-stimulating pills.
- Ask your health professional for advice if you think you need a different pill or insulin to suit your shift pattern.

Driving

You can obtain a license for most types of vehicle when you have diabetes. This means that, along with other motorists, you are responsible for your own safety and that of other people on the road. For this reason, it is very important to take precautions to avoid low blood sugar while driving. If you do become hypoglycemic at the wheel, know how to avoid endangering yourself or other people. You should also make sure that your vision is good enough to drive safely (see p.195).

Diabetes may affect driving performance if you have any long-term complications that can impair sensory or motor function. Examples of these complications include diabetic eye disease (retinopathy), nerve damage (neuropathy), kidney disease (nephropathy), cardiovascular disease, peripheral vascular disease, and stroke.

As the presence and extent of these factors vary from person to person, the Canadian Diabetes Association (CDA) maintains the following position on Driving and Licensing: People with diabetes have the right to be assessed for a license to drive a motor vehicle on an individual basis in accordance with Canadian Diabetes Association guidelines for private and commercial driving.

Motor vehicle licensing authorities can require licensed drivers to be examined for their medical fitness to drive. You should not have difficulty

---

My experience

"I don't want to feel different, but some people are ignorant about diabetes and think I have some major disability that will prevent me from doing my job properly." SHELLEY

COMMENT Your colleagues may know little about diabetes, or they may know someone with diabetes and expect you to be the same. Taking time to explain how diabetes affects you as an individual will dispel misconceptions and lessen some of your own frustrations.

---

obtaining and maintaining an operator's license if you:
- manage your diabetes properly
- are able to recognize and treat the early symptoms of hypoglycemia
- do not have complications that may interfere with your ability to drive.

In most Canadian jurisdictions, your doctor is required to report anyone he or she considers unfit to drive. For example, with regard to diabetes, this could include someone who is newly diagnosed and is just beginning to use insulin, someone who is not recognizing the early symptoms of hypoglycemia (unawareness), someone who has just experienced a severe hypoglycemic reaction, or someone who is not managing diabetes responsibly.

In June 2003, the CDA published Clinical Practice Guidelines for Diabetes and Private and Commercial Driving.

Safety at the wheel

Driving while you are hypoglycemic is as dangerous as driving under the influence of drugs or alcohol. If you know that you are hypoglycemic or

Myth OR TRUTH?

MYTH
When you're on vacation, you can also take a break from your diabetes.

TRUTH
You may be more relaxed about food and drink on vacation, but you can't afford to forget about your diabetes—unusual routines and heat can cause your blood glucose level to change more than usual. You will need to keep an eye on your blood glucose level and perhaps adjust your insulin or pill doses to prevent it from getting too high or low. You should also take swift action if you get a vacation stomach upset as well as taking particular care to look after your feet.

My experience

"When I'm packing to go away, it really annoys me that I have to leave space in my suitcase for all my diabetes equipment. I know I need it, but I still resent it!" JOE

COMMENT When you have diabetes you may have extra luggage, but it is worth being well prepared because you may not be able to obtain the equipment you need while you are away.

have engaged in behavior that is likely to lead to hypoglycemia, avoid driving—ask a friend to take you instead, or take a taxi.

You are at risk of low blood sugar only if you take insulin-stimulating pills or insulin injections. In both cases, you need to take the following precautions when you drive.

- Always test your blood glucose before you drive, to check that it is at a safe level.
- Test your blood glucose level at least every 2 hours during a long trip.
- Keep supplies of food and drink to treat low blood sugar (see p.106) close by (not in the trunk of the car).
- Carry identification.

If you have a hypoglycemic episode while driving, pull over immediately, stop the car, and treat yourself. Make it clear that you do not intend to continue until you have recovered by taking your keys out of the ignition and moving to the passenger seat. Do not drive again until your blood glucose level is above 4 millimoles per liter and you feel well.

If you know you do not experience clear warning signs during a hypoglycemic episode, you will need to be much stricter about stopping to test your blood glucose frequently or by traveling with people who will quickly recognize if you are starting to become hypoglycemic.

Vacations and travel

When you are away from home, whether on vacation or for business reasons, a different environment or routine is likely to have an effect on your diabetes management. There are a number of practicalities to consider before you go. Long-distance travel, changes in temperature, and different foods, drinks, or activities can all affect your blood glucose. The better you can plan ahead and anticipate any potential problems, the more enjoyable and successful your trip will be.

Before you go

Check that you will be insured for any diabetes-related problems while you are away. Make sure that your travel insurance includes preexisting conditions such as diabetes and that you are covered for any hospital stay and for your return trip.

Wherever you're going, you will need to take more than enough diabetes equipment and medication for the trip. Even if you are traveling within Canada, it can be difficult to get hold of replacement equipment or medication at short notice. Abroad, many pills, insulin, and blood-testing strips are named differently and may even be packaged in different sizes or strengths. Having plenty of your own supplies allows you to always stay in control of your treatment.

If you will be flying, make sure your insulin vials, pens, injectors, and pump are accompanied by a professionally printed pharmaceutical label identifying the medication. It is very important to keep some equipment with you in case your luggage is lost. Also, insulin can freeze in the hold of an aircraft, making it ineffective. Lancets can also be taken on board if they are capped and accompanied by a glucose meter that has the manufacturer's name embossed on the meter. It's a good idea to put some supplies in a traveling companion's hand luggage, too, in case yours is lost.

Before you travel, find out what types of food will be available at your destination so that you can take any extra foods you may need with you. Bear in mind that traveling across time zones can affect your blood glucose level, your eating pattern, and the timing of your treatment. Thinking in advance about when you expect to fly and arrive, and when your meal times are likely to be, will help you plan what measures to take and what food to carry with you in case there is none available when you need it.

CHECKING IN FOR A FLIGHT
When you check in, let airline staff know that you have diabetes medication and equipment in your hand luggage. If necessary show them your letter from your health professional.

TRAVELING LONG DISTANCES

• If you travel west, your day will be longer, so your medication will stop working effectively before the end of your day. Consequently, you may need an extra dose of your pills or insulin with an additional meal.

• If you travel east, your day will be shorter, so your medication will still be working, even though your body is telling you it is the end of the day. In this situation, you may need to eat more to compensate.

When you pack, include the following:
• Insulin or pills—at least double your normal supply; extra prescriptions.
• Blood glucose monitoring meter, lancets, and strips.
• Cold pack or thermos to store insulin.
• Hypoglycemia treatments.
• Food supplies.
• Identification.
• Information about how to manage your diabetes when you are ill.
• Your physician's contact details.
• Insurance details.

Looking after your equipment and medication

All your equipment and medicines should be stored in a cool, dry place. Unopened insulin bottles, cartridges,

HEAT AND DEHYDRATION
Hot weather can cause dehydration, as can a high blood glucose level. A combination of the two will you make you feel very ill. In a hot climate, you should drink plenty of water or other sugar-free fluids, and monitor your blood glucose level regularly.

or disposable injection devices should all be kept in a refrigerator (at a temperature of 2–8°C/36–47°F).
If you don't have access to one at your destination or if you are traveling a long distance, you will need to use a cold pack or thermos to store your insulin. If you are flying, make sure that you keep your insulin with you in your hand luggage because it can freeze in the hold of a plane.

The insulin you are currently using will be safe at a room temperature of up to 25°C (77°F) for up to a month, provided you keep it out of direct sunlight. At higher temperatures, you will need to keep it on a cold pack or in a cooler, thermos, water, or wrapped in cool cloths. In cool climates, you will need to keep your insulin above 2°C (36°F), either on your person or using a thermos.

Crossing time zones

When you are traveling across time zones, blood glucose testing every few hours is essential to find out whether you need any extra medication or food. You may find that your blood glucose level is erratic for 24 hours.

Hypoglycemia is always a concern when crossing time zones but, because you are probably using less energy than usual while traveling, the risk is somewhat reduced. If you are feeling excited or stressed, the hormones you produce will also have the effect of elevating your blood glucose level. If, during the trip, your level is a little higher than you would like, you can rectify this when you arrive at your destination. Traveling across time zones is less problematic if you are taking rapid-acting insulin analogue (see pp.84–85) or pills (see pp.76–81). If you are not using this type of medication and you anticipate problems when traveling, ask your health professional whether a change in medication would benefit you.

While you are away

Hot weather increases your circulation, speeding up the rate at which insulin or pills are absorbed into your bloodstream. (This can also happen if you have a massage or use hot jacuzzis, spas, or tanning beds.) Therefore, if you take insulin or insulin-stimulating pills, heat can make you susceptible to hypoglycemia. You may need to reduce your dose or have extra carbohydrate snacks or eat more carbohydrate at mealtimes to make low blood sugar less likely.

If you become very cold, for example while skiing, your circulation will slow down. As a result, your insulin or pills may take longer than usual to work. Wearing warm clothes and being physically active are likely to counteract this, so your blood glucose level shouldn't rise too high. Whatever the weather, it's important to keep testing your blood glucose to deal with any temperature-related problems.

While you are away, you may want to experiment with new foods, drinks, and activities. Again, testing will enable you to find out what effects these may have on your blood glucose and help you keep it within the recommended range. To avoid stomach upsets, which may cause your blood glucose level to rise, be careful about what you consume. Eat food that has been cooked properly and not left standing, drink bottled mineral or spring water, and eat only well-washed salad and peeled fruit.

If you take part in any strenuous physical activity, remember that it may affect your blood glucose many hours later, so you need to know how to prevent hypoglycemia in these circumstances (see pp.56–59).

Don't forget to look after your feet. It's all too easy to scrape your foot in the ocean, or to develop blisters when you're sightseeing or on hot sand, and not notice any injury. Never wear new shoes for the first time on vacation—take your most comfortable shoes. Also, never go barefoot, even on the beach. Keeping your feet protected by footwear at all times will reduce the risk of injury. Check your feet frequently and take action if necessary (see pp.128–130).

> If you become very cold, for example while skiing, your circulation will slow down. As a result, your insulin or pills may take longer than usual to work.

My experience

"I have traveled the world 3 times, lived in the desert, gone backpacking, ice climbing, and bicycling. You can do whatever you want—just manage your diabetes as you go along." JOE

COMMENT Diabetes does not have to prevent you from going anywhere you want to go or doing any activity you'd like. Planning ahead and thinking carefully about how you will manage your diabetes in different circumstances will ensure that your trip is successful.

"I always had the fear that no man would ever want to marry me because I had diabetes. But I told my husband-to-be when I met him, and it never put him off!" SOPHIE

COMMENT You may be wary of telling a new partner that you have diabetes, especially if you expect him or her to react badly. However, it's important to be honest from the start, even if you expect the worst—you could be surprised by the positive response you receive.

TALKING TO EACH OTHER
Diabetes can give rise to conflicting emotions within a relationship, often due to love, concern, stress, or fear. Sharing your feelings with your partner, ideally at times when neither of you is feeling pressured, will help you understand each other's point of view.

Sex and relationships

Diabetes has implications not only for you, but also for your partner and needs to be considered when you have sex, both in terms of the effect of sexual activity on your blood glucose level and the possibility of pregnancy. Reliable contraception is all-important when you are female and have diabetes, because you need very good blood glucose control before you conceive and during pregnancy.

Diabetes can also affect sexual function, most commonly in men, but also in women.

Finding ways of involving your partner if he or she wants to feel included can help alleviate concerns when they arise. For example, you might want to take your partner to your annual diabetes checkup so that he or she can gain a better understanding of any treatment you need. There may, however, be aspects of your diabetes care that you prefer to manage on your own. Be honest with your partner if this is how you feel—it is your diabetes, your health, and your decision as to how you deal with it.

Blood glucose control

Because sexual activity can use up a lot of energy, it should be treated in the same way as other types of physical activity (see pp.56–58). There are also a number of additional practicalities to consider. If you take insulin or insulin-stimulating pills, there is a risk that sex, like any form of strenuous activity, could cause hypoglycemia. Testing your blood glucose level before you have sex and again a few hours later will help you gauge the effect and decide whether you need to take any measures to prevent low blood sugar. You may find that you need to either

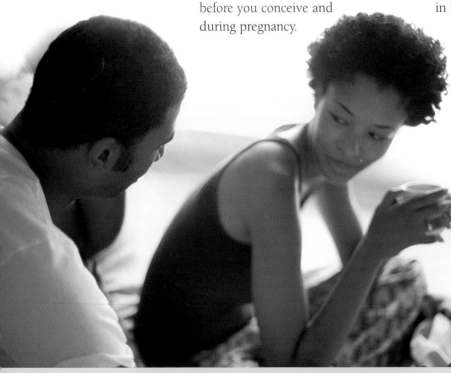

reduce your insulin dose beforehand or eat more to keep your blood glucose level within the ideal range.

Keep some high-carbohydrate snacks or drinks on hand, so that if you have a hypoglycemic episode, you can deal with it quickly (see p.106). Remember that your blood glucose level can fall several hours after physical activity, so you should be prepared. Your partner may need to give you a glucagon injection if you become too hypoglycemic to take action yourself.

Contraception

When you have diabetes, it is extremely important that pregnancy is planned, because good blood glucose control is essential from the moment of conception (see pp.138–147 for more information on diabetes and pregnancy). You can use any method of contraception, so it's important to choose the one that will be most reliable for you.

Oral contraceptive pills contain low doses of hormones. These may have a slight effect on your blood glucose level, but they are among the most reliable forms of contraception and are completely safe to take if you have diabetes. If your blood glucose level fluctuates a lot while taking an oral contraceptive, you can adjust your insulin or pills to compensate.

Sexual function

Problems with sexual function or performance are not unique to people with diabetes. However, erectile

Q Does having diabetes mean that sex can never be spontaneous?

A You should test your blood glucose level before having sex, as with before any physical activity, but there are always occasions when you want to be spontaneous. In general, having spontaneous sex (without testing beforehand) at times when you know that your blood glucose level will be low, is unwise. If you haven't tested your blood glucose level before having sex, have a high-glucose snack directly after sex and test your blood glucose, too.

dysfunction (see pp.213–215) is recognized as a complication of diabetes in men. Sexual function has been less widely researched in women, but it is thought that diabetes can affect a woman's sexual response. Vaginal dryness is a fairly common complaint, while some women might find sex painful, lose interest in sex, or be unable to achieve an orgasm as they used to.

Problems with sexual performance may have physical or psychological roots. If you are experiencing difficulties, you could talk to your health professional about treatment options. If there is a physical cause, you may be offered treatments such as vaginal lubricants if you are a woman, or drugs that stimulate your erection if you are a man who is experiencing difficulty with this. Some drugs may also be useful for women, although this form of treatment is still being researched. Counseling can help you deal with psychological issues.

When you have diabetes, it is extremely important that pregnancy is planned, because good blood glucose control is essential from the moment of conception.

Looking after yourself

When you have diabetes, there are aspects of your health that need special attention. For example, your feet should be checked daily. Because common illnesses can affect diabetes control, it's important to take steps to keep your blood glucose level in the target range and help speed up your recovery. Being admitted to the hospital may also disrupt your diabetes management; knowing what to do in this situation is also important.

Foot care

Over time, diabetes can have an impact on the efficiency of your blood circulation and nervous system, which can affect many areas of the body. Your feet are particularly susceptible to problems caused by poor circulation and nerve damage because they are farthest from your heart, and the main nerves in your legs are very long. You are, therefore, more susceptible to foot ulcers and other injuries, which can become infected and lead to serious problems. Also, because nerve damage can cause numbness in such extremities, you may not experience the soreness that would normally alert you to any injuries.

In extreme cases, an injury may take a long time to heal or can even lead to your foot or leg being amputated. This is why your feet and circulation are examined at your annual checkup (see p.26). In between checkups, you can take

good care of your feet yourself by checking them every day. Most importantly, you can help prevent injuries by never walking barefoot, not even in your own home and particularly not when you are in unfamiliar surroundings. Wear something on your feet indoors and out, and always on a beach to avoid burning your feet on hot sand.

Your daily routine

Wash and dry your feet thoroughly every day, and apply an unperfumed moisturizing cream afterward if your feet are dry, but don't put lotion between your toes. Check the top and sides of your feet carefully, looking for any tender, bruised, or hard, cracked, or callused skin, and the beginnings of blisters or corns.

Check the soles of your feet, too. (If this is hard for you to do, ask someone to help you.) Cut your toenails when you need to. However, if you know that you have reduced

DEALING WITH ILLNESS
Common illnesses, such as colds and flu, cause your body to produce the hormones epinephrine (adrenaline) and cortisol to fight infection. This can raise your blood glucose level. For this reason, it's important to monitor your blood glucose more frequently when you are ill.

feeling or circulation in your feet, check with your health professional that it is still alright for you to cut your own nails. If you can't bend to cut your nails, or they are too thick to cut, ask someone to help you.

Dealing with problems

Although you can treat some minor foot problems yourself, keep in mind that some fairly ordinary foot conditions, such as corns and hard skin, require the attention of a health professional.

■ **MINOR PROBLEMS** Athlete's foot can be treated at home with a fungal powder or cream. Keep the skin clean and dry, especially between your toes.

If you have a small blister, don't pop it, and avoid putting pressure on it. If the blister pops, cover it with a piece of gauze and tape, and keep checking it to make sure it heals.

Plantar warts will normally go away without treatment in time, but they may cause an imbalance of pressure

on your feet, especially if your nerves have been affected. Being assessed by a health professional will give you the information you need and enable you to treat them appropriately.

■ **WHEN TO GET HELP** Most other foot problems require professional care, so you need to contact your health professional if you develop any of the following conditions:

• Corns—never treat these yourself, either by cutting them or rubbing

> **Q** Why all the fuss about my feet just because I have diabetes? Surely I would be able to tell if there were something wrong?

> **A** Sometimes foot problems start because the nerves supplying the feet have been damaged. If this applies to you, you may not feel a small injury or notice a problem developing until it becomes serious. The only way to tell if anything is wrong is to check your feet all over every day. If you can't do this yourself, ask someone to do it for you.

You can help prevent injuries by never walking barefoot, not even in your own home, and particularly not when you are in unfamiliar surroundings.

LOOKING AFTER YOUR FEET

A good foot-care regimen will help you keep your feet healthy and enable you to notice potential problems early on. Carry out this procedure every day, allowing plenty of time to thoroughly check your feet for injuries and problems.

1 Wash your feet daily in warm water, using a mild soap. Avoid soaking your feet for more than 10 minutes, however, because this can dry out the skin.

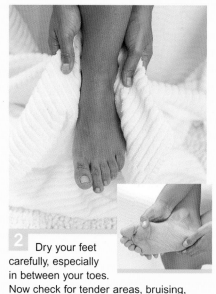

2 Dry your feet carefully, especially in between your toes. Now check for tender areas, bruising, and cuts or hard or cracked skin on the top and on the soles of your feet.

3 Trim your toenails when you need to. Cut them to the shape of and level with the end of your toe. Don't cut them too short and don't stick sharp instruments down the side of a nail.

4 Apply an unperfumed moisturizing cream to your feet, but not between your toes. Focus on hard skin on your soles.

them, and never use medicated corn plasters or dressings.

- Burns or injuries.
- A sore area that isn't healing.
- An ingrown toenail.
- Bruising or discolored areas on your feet with no apparent cause.
- Hard or cracked skin.
- New loss of feeling in any part of your foot—for example, if you can't feel a stone in your shoe.

It is important to get professional help if you can't look after your feet yourself and there is no one else to do it for you, or if you are concerned about your feet in any way, even if you think your worry is trivial.

Daily comfort

Don't wear tight or restrictive socks, stockings, or panty hose that rub or cramp your toes, and remember not to put your feet directly against a hot-water bottle, hot radiator, or heater, or near an open fire, since you may accidentally burn your feet if you can't feel the heat. Check your shoes daily to make sure there are no parts that are rubbing your feet, or sharp objects inside the shoe or sticking through the sole. Also, check the soles and tops of your shoes for uneven wear that may indicate particular areas of pressure on your feet.

When you become ill

In itself, having diabetes does not make you more susceptible to common illnesses than anyone else. But if your diabetes is poorly controlled and your blood glucose level is consistently high, you may pick up infections more easily or just feel ill. This is because bacteria and viruses thrive when your blood glucose is consistently above 10 millimoles per liter. Any illness can affect your diabetes, particularly if it lasts several days, or requires medical or hospital treatment. Blood glucose control can also affect the speed of your recovery.

The effect on your diabetes

Whatever type of diabetes you have, illness is likely to raise your blood glucose level. This is because part of your body's natural reaction to illness is to release more glucose into your bloodstream and to produce stress hormones such as epinephrine (adrenaline) and cortisol. These hormones make your natural or injected insulin less efficient, which can cause hyperglycemia, even if you are not eating anything.

One symptom of hyperglycemia is dehydration, which can be aggravated by a high body temperature. Therefore, a sudden, acute illness, such as food poisoning with vomiting and diarrhea, and its combined effects of high blood glucose, dehydration, and infection, can cause your diabetes to become seriously out of control and also affect other body processes.

If you have type 1 diabetes, this situation may result in diabetic ketoacidosis (see p.113). If you have type 2 diabetes, you might become severely dehydrated, which can

occasionally lead to coma (see p.113) Both require urgent hospital treatment. Set up a sick-day plan with your doctor now, before you need one.

Blood glucose control

You may not be ill very often, so it can be difficult to remember what effect illness has on your blood glucose level and how to respond. Next time you are ill, write down what action you take to control your blood glucose and keep your notes to refer to again if you need to.

When you are ill, there are two golden rules to remember:
● Test your blood glucose level at least every four hours.
● Continue taking your insulin or pills, even if you are not eating anything.

Your tests will tell you what effect your illness is having on your blood glucose level, while taking your pills or insulin will help combat the natural increase in blood glucose that illness causes. If you feel too ill to do blood glucose tests or even to think about your diabetes treatment, you need to ask a friend or family member to do it for you, or contact your health professional.

When you are ill, keeping your blood glucose level below 10 millimoles per liter will help your recovery. You may need to temporarily increase your dose of pills or insulin to achieve this, and you can reduce the dose again when you feel better. If you have a longer illness, particularly when you are

Myth OR TRUTH?

MYTH
If you are not able to eat when you're ill, you should stop taking your pills or insulin to prevent a hypoglycemic reaction.

TRUTH
Your body produces glucose even if you are not eating when you are ill, and may produce more to give your body extra energy to recover from illness. You need to continue or even increase your pills or insulin to keep your glucose level down.

Whatever type of diabetes you have, illness is likely to raise your blood glucose level.

COPING WITH ILLNESS

- Drink up to 16 cups (128 fl.oz/3.8 liters) of sugar-free fluids throughout the day.
- If you are not able to eat solid food for any reason, have milk, fruit juice, or soup at mealtimes.
- If you have type 1 diabetes, continue taking some insulin, even if you are not eating normally. Try to have food and drinks that appeal to you when ill.
- Check for ketones in your urine. If present, drink more water or sugar-free fluids.
- If you are vomiting and unable to keep food or drink down, or are simply not sure what to do, contact your health professional as soon as possible.

Drugs that you buy over the counter are safe to take when you have diabetes, although some may affect your blood glucose level.

confined to bed for weeks or months, keeping your blood glucose level within the normal range will help prevent complications from arising.

If your body is particularly sensitive to insulin, illness can occasionally cause hypoglycemia. If you have type 1 diabetes and experience a "honeymoon period"—a period of up to two years after being diagnosed with diabetes when your pancreas makes some insulin again—your body will be sensitive to insulin during this time. Children may also experience a lower blood glucose level when ill. In these circumstances, you may need to reduce your dose of pills or insulin, but be careful that this doesn't make your blood glucose level rise too high.

Eating and drinking

Eating and drinking gives your body energy to combat your illness and limits the effects of an illness on your diabetes. You may also need small amounts of drinks containing glucose. If you can't eat, a day or two without food will not matter too much, but drinking plenty of sugar-free fluids throughout the day is essential. This helps keep your temperature down and prevent dehydration if your blood glucose level is elevated.

Diarrhea and vomiting

Your body tries to get rid of anything it perceives as harmful, such as infected food, by expelling it from your system. Bouts of vomiting and diarrhea may be short-lived, but they can have a serious effect on your

diabetes within a few hours.

■ **TYPE 1 DIABETES** If you become hyperglycemic and dehydrated as a result of prolonged vomiting and diarrhea, and you are not able to keep any food or fluids down, your body might develop ketones in large quantities. Ketones make you even more nauseated because they irritate your stomach, and they also affect the acid balance of your blood. If this happens, your organs are unable to function properly, which could lead to unconsciousness and even death. This condition is known as diabetic ketoacidosis (see p.113).

You can prevent diabetic ketoacidosis and serious illness by always taking your insulin, even if you are not eating, are being sick, or simply don't feel like injecting. You need to test your urine or blood for ketones using dipsticks or a blood glucose meter in order to assess the seriousness of your condition. If you have ketones, or if you have diarrhea and vomiting that continues for more than 2–3 hours, contact your health professional. You may need to be treated in the hospital.

■ **TYPE 2 DIABETES** You are unlikely to develop diabetic ketoacidosis if you have diarrhea and vomiting, but your blood glucose level can still rise extremely high and you can become very dehydrated, which can lead to a coma (a condition known as hyperglycemic nonketotic hyperosmolar state, see p.113). If you are unable to take your pills (if you have them) or to keep any fluids down, contact your health professional at once, since you may need treatment for your dehydration, either at home or in the hospital.

Over-the-counter medicines

Drugs that you buy over the counter are safe to use if you have diabetes, although some may affect your blood glucose level. Cough syrup, for example, may contain a lot of sugar, but since you only take a teaspoonful or two of syrup in a single dose, the effect on your blood glucose will be minimal. Ideally, ask your pharmacist to recommend a low-sugar product.

Long-term drug treatments

If you are prescribed drugs to treat a condition other than your diabetes, these might affect your blood glucose level. If a range of drugs is available to treat your condition, your physician will choose the one that has the least effect on your blood glucose. If there is only one drug treatment your physician can prescribe and this is likely to affect your blood glucose, the type or dose of insulin or pills you take for your diabetes may need to change.

High blood pressure

Certain pills used to treat high blood pressure, including thiazide diuretics such as hydrochlorthiazide and beta blockers such as propranolol, can affect your blood glucose level. High blood pressure can be difficult to

---

"When I'm ill, I check my blood glucose every 2–3 hours and do urine tests. If I have ketones, I take more insulin. If I am vomiting, I sip sugary drinks and drink water to flush out ketones." SHELLEY

COMMENT Developing a procedure that you can follow whenever you are ill will help you stay in control of your diabetes and avoid potential problems. When you have type 1 diabetes, testing for ketones is particularly important to identify when the illness is becoming serious.

treat when you have diabetes, so you might need two or three different types of pills in combination to keep it under control. If the pills you take affect your blood glucose it is still extremely important to take them, because reducing high blood pressure is just as important as lowering blood glucose in the prevention of long-term complications (see pp.206–208). If you start new medication, monitoring your blood glucose level to assess its effect will tell you whether you need to change your dose or type of pills or insulin to compensate.

TAKING DIABETES PILLS
When you are ill, you should keep taking your diabetes pills and/or insulin—even if you are not eating—to combat the effect of illness on your blood glucose.

Steroid treatment

Steroids, such as prednisolone or dexamethasone, can have a significant effect on your blood glucose. These are used to reduce inflammation, and to treat a variety of different conditions including:

• Chronic lung conditions: chronic obstructive pulmonary disease (COPD), asthma.

• Chronic bowel conditions: Crohn's disease, ulcerative colitis.

• Joint inflammation: rheumatoid arthritis.

• Cancer.

Steroid treatment is also used after organ transplantation to reduce the possibility of rejection. Steroid pills or injections increase your blood glucose level, and you will need to increase the dose of your pills or insulin to compensate, even if you are only taking steroids for a short time. Even if you don't have diabetes, steroids can increase your blood glucose level and cause diabetes to develop. Taking steroids via an inhaler or a skin patch will not affect your blood glucose in the same way that pills and injections do.

Taking a combination of pills

When you have diabetes, you may find yourself taking five or more different pills and perhaps insulin injections, too, to control not only your blood glucose but also your blood pressure and blood fat levels. If you have other conditions, such as diabetes complications, you may

Steroid pills or injections increase your blood glucose level and you will need to increase the dose of your pills or insulin to compensate.

Q I have had pills for my blood pressure for some time. Now I've been given another type to take as well. I don't feel any different—do I really need to take both?

A Many people need more than one type of pill for good blood pressure control. Most pills are prescribed on a trial basis—you need to take them for a while to find out whether they work for you. Although taking lots of pills may seem like a chore, the treatment you receive is aimed at preventing health problems in the future, so you need to persevere if you are to benefit in the long term.

need to take even more. However many pills are prescribed, you should take them all as instructed—even if they don't seem to make a difference to the way you feel. Your treatment is designed to keep you healthy in the long term. If you are concerned about the number of pills you take, ask your physician or pharmacist to check regularly that they are all still necessary.

Going into the hospital

If you are admitted to the hospital, whether as a result of your diabetes (if you develop diabetic ketoacidosis, for example, or you have a diabetes complication) or for something unrelated, such as a broken leg, you will need to make decisions about your diabetes care with hospital staff.

In the hospital, your treatment, mealtimes, and blood glucose testing routine will not be the same as at home. To enable your body to recover normally, your blood glucose level should be less than 10 millimoles per liter most of the time. To achieve this, your pills or insulin should be given at the correct time in relation to your meals, and your usual dose of medication may even need to be increased. If you need snacks between meals or at bedtime, these should be made available, or you might keep some supplies yourself.

You may need to let staff know when you need to test your blood glucose or need your pills or insulin, because they won't be as familiar with your diabetes as you are. You may be able to do your own tests and take your own medication, or ask for them when you need them. If you are concerned, discuss your diabetes with senior staff.

If you are unable to eat or drink for more than a few hours, such as for surgery for which you need an empty stomach, or if you are unconscious, hospital staff will take over your diabetes care. Your blood glucose will be carefully controlled using an insulin infusion and glucose drip, which are inserted into your vein. The rate at which insulin enters your bloodstream is adjusted according to your blood glucose level, which is measured every hour.

As soon as you are eating properly, the glucose drip and insulin infusion will be removed. You can then resume your normal diabetes treatment. Ideally, you will have the first dose of your usual treatment shortly before the drip and infusion are removed to make sure that your blood glucose doesn't rise as a result of the insulin supply suddenly being removed before your usual treatment has had time to work.

When you are discharged

During your hospital stay, changes may have been made to your diabetes pills or insulin type or regimen. It is important that you know about any new medication, when to take it, and how. If you don't understand why it has changed or what effect it might have, speak to a health professional before you leave. If you have been far less active in the hospital than normal and you take insulin-stimulating pills or insulin, you might be at risk of hypoglycemia when you resume your normal activities, so discuss whether the discharge dose will still be right for you when you get home.

Outpatient visits

If you go into the hospital as an outpatient, such as for minor surgery, you may be asked not to eat or drink for several hours beforehand. If you take insulin-stimulating pills or insulin, and are unable to balance these with food, you will be at risk of hypoglycemia. To prevent this, reduce your dose before you begin to fast and test your blood glucose regularly while you are not eating or drinking and during the procedure. If you cannot do your own testing for any reason, staff will need to take over.

When you have diabetes, most procedures take place early in the day so that you can resume your normal treatment as quickly as possible.

Practical tips

PREPARING FOR A HOSPITAL PROCEDURE

- Make sure you know exactly when your surgery or investigation is taking place and that hospital staff know you have diabetes.
- Ask for advice on what to do about your diabetes treatment if you have to fast before the procedure.
- Test your blood glucose regularly before and after the procedure, or ask staff.
- Take your first meal and medication to the hospital for use after the procedure; and your hypoglycemia treatment, if you take insulin or insulin-stimulating pills.

Women's health

If you are a woman with diabetes, it is important to know how your hormones and common female complaints can affect your blood glucose level. If you plan to have children, it is essential to prepare well before you conceive and to manage your diabetes strictly during pregnancy to safeguard your own and your baby's health and to maximize your chances of a trouble-free labor and delivery. If you develop gestational diabetes, you will need to take similar care to manage this condition.

Practical tips

AVOIDING MENSTRUAL HIGHS AND LOWS

- Try to stick to your healthy eating plan, even if you feel like eating less healthy foods.
- Limit your salt intake, since it causes water retention.
- Cut back on alcohol, caffeine, and chocolate; these can affect your blood glucose level as well as your mood.
- Eat at regular intervals to avoid swings in your blood glucose level.
- Do some regular physical activity—being active may improve your mood and make it easier to control your blood glucose level.

Female hormones

The female hormones estrogen and progesterone are produced by the ovaries. Together, these hormones regulate your menstrual cycle and maintain a pregnancy.

Your menstrual cycle

During your menstrual cycle, levels of estrogen and progesterone in your body rise and fall. At the beginning of your cycle, estrogen causes the lining of the uterus to thicken. If conception does not occur, more progesterone is produced to trigger the shedding of the uterine lining. You may find that these monthly hormonal fluctuations have an effect on your blood glucose level.

If you suspect that your menstrual cycle is affecting your blood glucose, test your blood glucose level frequently (four or more times a day) just before, during, and directly

after your period and record the results to help identify any regular pattern. If you find that your blood glucose level tends to rise just before your period, you could:

- Try fitting in some extra physical activity to bring your blood glucose level down.
- Avoid eating too many extra carbohydrates.
- Try increasing your insulin dose in the few days before your period is due.

If, on the other hand, your blood glucose is lower than normal and you have a tendency to experience hypoglycemia more often, you could:

- Try increasing your intake of carbohydrate-containing foods.
- Reduce your insulin dose in the few days before your period.

The way in which your menstrual periods affect your blood glucose level is likely to remain fairly constant from one cycle to the next; therefore,

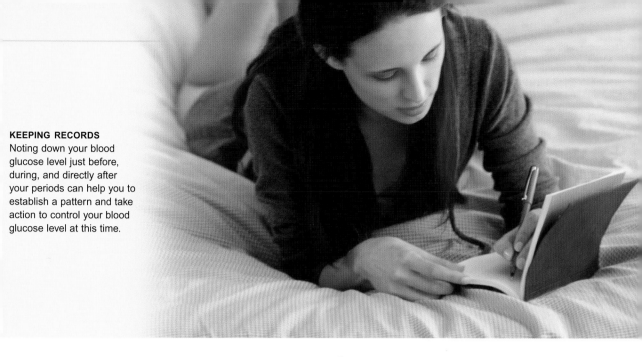

even if you change your diabetes treatment, over time you should be able to work out how to keep your blood glucose balanced throughout your monthly cycle.

Menopause

Many changes occur in a woman's body during menopause, but these will not necessarily affect your diabetes and its treatment. However, you may find that some symptoms of menopause are similar to those that occur when you have a high or low blood glucose level. If you do feel hot or shaky, or start sweating, testing your blood glucose level can help you decide whether you need to treat your diabetes at this time.

Hormone replacement therapy (HRT), which relieves menopausal symptoms, is controversial. Ask your health professional whether taking HRT would be right for you.

Cystitis and yeast

Inflammation of the bladder lining, which is known as cystitis, and a fungal infection of the vagina, known as yeast, are conditions that commonly affect women. Cystitis is generally caused by a bacterial infection and causes frequent and painful urination. Yeast develops when the fungus *Candida albicans*, which can occur naturally in the vagina, grows more rapidly than usual. Yeast can cause unpleasant itching and a discharge. Cystitis and yeast can occur more frequently when you have diabetes because a slightly raised blood glucose level provides the type of environment in which bacteria and fungi thrive. An infection can cause your blood glucose level to rise even further (see p.131). If you think you may have cystitis or yeast, see your doctor. Treatment for both of these conditions are available from your doctor or pharmacist.

Cystitis and yeast can occur more frequently when you have diabetes because a slightly elevated blood glucose level provides the type of environment in which bacteria and fungi thrive.

Practical tips

GIVING YOUR BABY THE BEST START

- As for any woman wishing to conceive, you should take a daily dose of folic acid for 3 months before you conceive and during the first 4 months of pregnancy. This improves cell growth and helps to guard against spina bifida and other rare spinal cord defects in your baby.

- Avoid eating pâté, raw shellfish, foods that contain raw eggs, and unpasteurized food, such as certain types of soft or blue-veined cheeses, since these may cause infections that can harm your baby.

- Cut out alcohol and cigarettes, and cut down on caffeine.

Pregnancy

Careful planning is very important when it comes to pregnancy and diabetes. Looking after your diabetes throughout your pregnancy and attending prenatal appointments will maximize your chances of having a healthy baby and as few problems as possible. Unless you have gestational diabetes (see pp.144–145), your diabetes will affect your pregnancy (and vice versa) right from the start.

Planning your pregnancy

Having diabetes doesn't make it more or less likely that you will be able to become pregnant, but it does increase the risk of you and your baby having problems. A high blood glucose level, that is an A1C level above 7 percent (see pp.66–67), around the time you conceive and in the first eight weeks of pregnancy, can affect your baby's development. This is why it is so important to plan your pregnancy carefully so that you know that your diabetes is under control when you conceive, and avoid accidental pregnancy by using a reliable method of contraception (see p.127).

If you want to have a baby, your health professional will be able to advise you on your blood glucose control, perform blood tests, check your health in general, and make any necessary referrals. In particular, you will need to have your eyes checked for diabetic retinopathy (see pp.190–194) because, if left untreated, this can worsen during pregnancy.

Before you conceive, you will need to check your blood glucose level at least three to four times a day and make sure that the majority of your tests are in the range of 4–7 millimoles per liter or less. You may need to work toward this by adjusting your insulin, pills, food intake, and activity level. It may be necessary to adjust your insulin dose to bring your blood glucose level under tight control. If this is difficult, or causes lots of hypoglycemic episodes, you may need to change your insulin regimen—for example, from twice-daily injections to a four-times-a-day regimen. More frequent injections will enable you to fit your insulin dose to your glucose level more accurately. See pp.90–95 for information on adjusting insulin doses and regimens.

If you take pills to control your diabetes, you may need to take insulin injections instead to achieve the control you need before becoming pregnant. When you do become pregnant you will certainly need to switch to insulin, because pills for diabetes may be harmful to your baby. You should be able to revert to your pills once your baby is born if they continue to control your blood glucose. Your health care team will help determine what is best for you and your baby as your pregnancy progresses.

Once your blood glucose is well controlled, your A1C level should be checked to confirm that it is 7 percent or less, so that when you

ROUTINE PRENATAL TESTS

Prenatal care starts as soon as you know that you are pregnant and is essential to ensure that the pregnancy is progressing well and that your diabetes is as well controlled as possible. You will have several routine tests at regular intervals throughout your pregnancy.

TEST	WHEN	REASON
A1C	Every 1–2 months	To check that your blood glucose level is tightly controlled, to make sure that your baby can grow and develop normally.
Retinal examination	During the first trimester, then as needed	To look for signs of diabetic retinopathy (see pp.192–193), which can develop or worsen during pregnancy.
Ultrasound scan	Every 1–2 months	To assess the development and growth of your baby and detect any abnormalities, using an image produced by sound waves.
Blood pressure	Every visit	To check for raised blood pressure, which increases the risk of pre-eclampsia (p.142).
Urine test	Every visit	To check for the presence of ketones, which can harm your baby.
Fetal monitoring	Every visit	To check your baby's heartbeat and movements.
Blood test for neural tube defects	At 16–18 weeks	To detect severe neural tube defects in your baby, which can cause disorders including spina bifida.
Amniocentesis	(Optional) at 18 weeks	To test for genetic abnormalities.

If your blood glucose level is high, your baby's will be, too. This is because glucose can cross your placenta into your baby's bloodstream but insulin cannot.

conceive, your baby will have the best chance of growing and developing normally.

ACE inhibitor pills for controlling blood pressure cannot be taken during pregnancy. Your health professional will be able to suggest alternatives.

While you are pregnant

Good diabetes control is crucial while you are pregnant, both for your baby's and your own health. If your blood glucose level is high, your baby's will be, too. This is because glucose can cross your placenta into your baby's bloodstream but insulin cannot. If your baby's glucose level is high, he or she will have to produce more insulin to lower it, which in turn causes extra glucose to be stored in your baby's body, causing faster than normal growth. As a result, you are more likely to experience a difficult labor and delivery and your baby may have problems with

HYPOGLYCEMIA DURING PREGNANCY

- Eat carbohydrate-containing foods regularly throughout the day.
- Test your blood glucose level at least 4 times a day and adjust your insulin according to the results.
- Sometimes the symptoms of hypoglycemia change during pregnancy, so if you have an unusual symptom, check your blood glucose right away—it could be a sign of low blood sugar.
- Keep glucose pills, a glucose drink, or dextrose gel with you at all times to use as soon as you feel the symptoms coming on.
- Tell your partner, a friend, or a colleague at work that hypoglycemia could occur, and if possible, show him or her how to give you a glucagon injection (see p.109), should you lose consciousness.

breathing and could experience hypoglycemia after birth.

If you have type 1 diabetes, another reason to keep your blood glucose level regulated during pregnancy is to prevent ketones from forming (see p.113). Ketones can be extremely harmful to your baby and, in rare situations, can even be fatal to your baby. Ketones can form during pregnancy even if your blood glucose level is not high enough to give you symptoms, so it is vital that you increase your insulin dose as soon as your blood glucose level starts to rise.

Throughout your pregnancy, you need to keep your pre-meal blood glucose level between 3.8–5.2 millimoles per liter and, 2 hours after meals, at 5.0–6.6 millimoles per liter. You should also keep your A1C at 7 percent or below.

As your pregnancy progresses, you will need larger doses of insulin to keep your blood glucose well controlled. This is because your growing baby and the additional hormones your placenta produces increase your body's need for insulin. By the ninth month, your original dose of insulin may have doubled, tripled, or more. As soon as your baby is born, your body's insulin requirement will reduce and you will revert to a dose close to what you were taking before you became pregnant.

■ **MORNING SICKNESS** In the early weeks of pregnancy, you may feel nauseated at any time. If you feel sick in the morning, try having a drink or a plain cookie before you get up, and split

your morning dose of insulin so that you take some when you normally would and the rest later when you feel like eating. To combat queasiness at other times, eat regular snacks of plain cookies, crackers, or fruit.

If you are vomiting and can't keep food down, your health professional can prescribe pregnancy-safe medicines that prevent the vomiting and give you advice on your insulin regimen. If you are very ill and there is a risk that your body might be producing ketones, you may be admitted to the hospital.

■ **PRENATAL CARE** Your prenatal care is especially important when you have diabetes. Care by an interdisciplinary healthcare team prior to conception and during pregnancy minimizes both maternal and fetal risks. You will need to visit your diabetes health care team (composed of diabetes nurse educators, registered dietitians, obstetricians, and endocrinologists/internists) more frequently during your pregnancy.

At your visits, you will be able to discuss the results of your home tests and any problems you are having. For example, you may experience more frequent, sudden, and severe episodes of hypoglycemia, especially in the first three months of your pregnancy, when your body's need for insulin can fluctuate unpredictably.

■ **LOOKING AFTER YOURSELF** Eating a healthy diet, being physically active on a regular basis—a brisk daily walk, gentle jog (if you are used to it), or swimming—and avoiding alcohol and cigarettes will all increase your chances of a successful, comfortable pregnancy. You should not attempt to diet when you are pregnant because you need enough energy for both you and your baby.

If you become ill for any reason during your pregnancy, your blood glucose level will rise and you will need more insulin. You should monitor your blood glucose level as you would normally, and correct it with insulin as necessary (see p.94). You should also test your urine or blood for ketones twice a day, and contact your health professional right away if ketones are present.

Very occasionally, babies die during the last few weeks of pregnancy. This is a more common occurrence when you have diabetes, but is still very rare. The chances of it happening to you are reduced if your diabetes has

My experience

"I would say that someone with diabetes receives even better prenatal care than someone who doesn't have it—so just once, diabetes has its perks!" LOUISE

COMMENT Although you need more frequent clinic visits when you are pregnant, you tend to see the same people each time and have very detailed tests and attention—so it can make you feel extra special.

been very well controlled. If there is a risk to your baby, you may be offered an induction or cesarean section before your expected birth date.

■ **PLANNING THE BIRTH** Because you may need special care during labor, you will probably be advised to have your baby in a hospital rather than at home. Talk to your health professional in advance to find out the options that are available in your area and what you can expect to happen to you and your baby during the birth.

KEEPING ACTIVE
Regular physical activity helps prepare you for the physical demands of labor and speed recovery after the birth. Swimming is a particularly comfortable form of exercise when you are pregnant because your weight is supported by the water.

Giving birth

Your labor may start normally, if all has gone well with your pregnancy, or you may need to be induced or have a Caesarean section if problems have arisen. If labor is progressing normally, you may wish to monitor your own blood glucose level, or ask your partner to do it for you. You need to test at least once an hour to monitor the level. If you have been advised not to eat (in case you should need an emergency general anesthetic), you are more likely to have a hypoglycemic episode, so regular blood glucose testing will warn you of this. Make sure that you give all your test results to hospital staff for their records.

If labor lasts a long time or starts when your glucose level may be falling, such as when you have not eaten for some time, you will probably be given an intravenous glucose drip

Once your baby is separated from your placenta, his or her blood glucose level falls. For this reason, when your baby is born, a blood sample will be taken to check whether he or she is hypoglycemic.

POTENTIAL PREGNANCY PROBLEMS

Most pregnancies progress smoothly, but all pregnant women face potential problems. Having diabetes makes some problems more likely. Healthy eating, regular physical activity, and excellent blood glucose control all greatly reduce the risk of difficulties occurring.

PROBLEM	IMPLICATIONS
Worsening of diabetes complications	If you already have eye complications, they may worsen in pregnancy. Your eyes are checked as part of your prenatal care so that any problems can be treated early. Kidney problems before pregnancy can increase your risk of raised blood pressure, so this is also checked regularly.
Oversized baby	A high blood glucose level can cause your baby to grow at an increased rate (known as macrosomia). Excellent blood glucose control reduces the risk of macrosomia. If it occurs, your baby may need to be delivered early.
Polyhydramnios	If your baby has a high blood glucose level, he or she may produce more urine, which can lead to an excessive amount of amniotic fluid in the uterus. Polyhydramnios can cause premature labor.
Preeclampsia	If severe or left untreated, preeclampsia can lead to a potentially fatal disorder known as eclampsia that causes seizures and may bring on a coma. If you have high blood pressure, protein in your urine, and fluid retention in the last 3 months of pregnancy, you are likely to be monitored in the hospital until your baby is born, or if you are near your delivery date, labor may be induced.
Premature labor	If labor starts before the 37th week of pregnancy, or you are induced early, your baby may not be fully developed and may need special care when he or she is born.

to keep your blood glucose stable until your baby is born. You will also receive an infusion of insulin via a vein, and the amounts will be adjusted according to your blood glucose level (see p.135). Your baby's heart rate, movements, and position will be checked throughout your labor. You can expect to be offered the same pain relief choices as any other mother, depending on how your labor is progressing.

After your baby is born

Once your baby is separated from your placenta, his or her blood glucose level falls. For this reason, when your baby is born, a blood sample will be taken to check whether he or she is hypoglycemic. If your baby has been born early but is the right size for a full-term pregnancy, there is a danger that his or her lungs may not be fully developed. As a result, your baby's breathing will also be carefully checked and, if necessary, he or she will be helped to breathe at first.

If all is well, you should be able to feed your baby immediately, although he or she may also need a glucose injection or bottle-feed to increase a low blood glucose level. If your baby

is seriously hypoglycemic or is having difficulty breathing, he or she may be moved to a special care baby unit to be closely monitored. In some hospitals, babies born to mothers with diabetes are routinely taken to a special care unit for observation immediately after birth.

After the delivery of your placenta, your need for insulin reduces suddenly and if you were receiving an insulin infusion during labor, the dosage rate will be lowered immediately to prevent you from becoming hypoglycemic. Unless you have had a general anesthetic, you will be able to eat and drink soon after the birth. You should then be able to take over your blood glucose testing

BONDING WITH YOUR BABY
There is no reason why diabetes should keep you from bonding normally with your new baby—even if you miss out on immediate contact, once you are both settled, you can start to get to know each other.

My experience

"As soon as Sam was born, my insulin requirements immediately returned to what they were before I was pregnant—literally for the first meal!" SOPHIE

COMMENT As soon as your placenta has been delivered, the effect of insulin-resisting estrogen hormones instantly disappears and your insulin requirement falls dramatically.

and insulin injections. You may be able to revert to pills if you were taking these before you were pregnant, unless you are breastfeeding. You cannot take pills for diabetes when you are breastfeeding, because they will affect your baby through your milk; you may need to continue taking insulin until your baby is weaned.

If you weren't taking insulin or pills before pregnancy, you may be able to revert to controlling your blood glucose through healthy eating and physical activity, in which case there are no special considerations with regard to breastfeeding.

> A growing baby and the hormones your body produces increase the demand for insulin. If your body is unable to meet this need, your blood glucose level will rise.

Gestational diabetes

It is not possible to determine whether you are susceptible to gestational diabetes before your first pregnancy until the condition becomes apparent—which is most likely to happen at about 28 weeks.

A growing baby and the hormones your body produces increase the demand for insulin. If your body is unable to meet this need, your blood glucose level will rise above normal. You will need a laboratory blood test

to diagnose gestational diabetes, and specialized prenatal care if you are found to have the condition.

Gestational diabetes usually disappears once your baby is born, but occasionally you may develop permanent type 1 or type 2 diabetes while you are pregnant. If you develop gestational diabetes, you have an increased risk of gestational diabetes in future pregnancies and of developing permanent type 2 diabetes in later years. You can reduce the likelihood of this happening by doing regular physical activity and keeping your weight in the recommended range (see p.46).

Diagnosis and treatment

The first sign of gestational diabetes is often a positive urine test for glucose. However, because it is common for pregnant women to have glucose in their urine, you will need to have one of two laboratory blood tests—a fasting or a random blood glucose test or an oral glucose tolerance test (see pp.20–21) to confirm your diagnosis. If you are diagnosed with gestational diabetes, you will receive the same prenatal care as any other woman with diabetes who is pregnant, to limit the risks to yourself and your baby (see pp.139–140).

Depending on your blood glucose level at diagnosis and the stage of your pregnancy, your initial treatment may involve adjusting your food intake. If you have been eating a lot of high-sugar foods, large meals containing lots of carbohydrate, or having sugary drinks, limiting these can make a big difference immediately to your blood glucose level. You should aim to keep your blood glucose level below 5.3 millimoles per liter before meals and, 2 hours after meals, below 6.7 millimoles per liter. Your health professional will show you how to test your own blood glucose level (see pp.62–75) to reveal how effective any changes to your eating habits have been.

If healthier eating is not enough to keep your blood glucose level in the recommended range, you will be offered insulin injections. Pills used to treat diabetes cannot be taken during pregnancy because there is a risk that they may harm your baby, whereas insulin is perfectly safe to use. You may need up to four injections each day to maintain tight control of your blood glucose level.

Birth and postnatal care

Because there is a possibility that your baby will need to be delivered by cesarean section or require care in a special unit once he or she is born, you will probably be advised to have your baby in the hospital. During labor, you may also need a glucose drip and an insulin infusion (see p.135) and more frequent monitoring of your blood pressure and your baby's movements and progress.

As soon as your baby is born, your body's need for insulin will reduce dramatically, so you will probably no longer require insulin treatment or need to check your blood glucose level. However, because there is a small risk of developing permanent type 1 or type 2 diabetes when you are pregnant, you will either have a continuing need for insulin treatment or have an oral glucose tolerance test six weeks after the birth of your baby to check that your body is still able to use glucose properly. For this reason, you may wish to continue to check your blood glucose level yourself for the few weeks before your formal glucose test. Whatever you do, you should be aware of diabetes-related symptoms (see pp.18–19) and see your health professional as soon as possible if you experience any of them.

Once you have had gestational diabetes, it is likely to recur in future pregnancies. You are also much more likely to develop type 2 diabetes later in life. Your risk is even greater if you are overweight, if other family members have type 2 diabetes, or if you are of African, Latin American, Aboriginal, or Asian descent. Once you have had gestational diabetes, you will need a fasting blood glucose test or oral glucose tolerance test at least every three years to check for type 2 diabetes.

You can delay or even prevent the onset of type 2 diabetes by keeping your weight in the recommended range for your height, doing regular physical activity, and eating healthily. If you experience any symptoms of diabetes, see your health professional.

Myth OR TRUTH?

MYTH
You cannot breastfeed if you have diabetes.

TRUTH Breastfeeding is an ideal start for your baby and having diabetes doesn't make it any less likely that you and your baby will be successful in this. You cannot take pills to control diabetes while you are breastfeeding, but there are other ways of managing your diabetes if you wish to breastfeed. Your health professional can advise you.

Life with a new baby

For any family, adjusting to life with a new baby can take time. Meals, sleep, and time to yourself or with your partner are all likely to be disrupted, which means that your diabetes routine will also be upset.

Although you can be a little less strict about your blood glucose control now that you are no longer pregnant, there are aspects of motherhood, such as breastfeeding, that may make a difference to your diabetes. Knowing what to expect as a new mother and how to manage your diabetes in these situations will help you through this period of adjustment.

Eating and drinking

Your mealtimes are likely to be irregular when you have a new baby, and this can affect your diabetes. If you go without food for too long and you take insulin or insulin-stimulating pills, you can become hypoglycemic or, if there are extended periods of time between your insulin doses, your blood glucose level may rise. You may find it useful to prepare or set aside some sandwiches, fruit, or cereal bars each day in case you are unable to eat or drink when planned. If your mealtimes are unpredictable and you take a ready-mixed insulin or are on a twice-a-day regimen, changing to a more flexible four-times-a-day system might suit your new lifestyle better.

Breastfeeding

When you breastfeed, you transfer energy to your baby through your milk. This means that you will need to eat at least an additional 50g of carbohydrate per day (see pp.35–36). If you take insulin, you may also need to reduce your dose to prevent hypoglycemia.

BREASTFEEDING
Breastfeeding is as suitable for your baby as for any other, and you have just the same chances of success as any other mother. If you take insulin, you may need to reduce your dose while you are breastfeeding, to prevent hypoglycemia.

When you are feeding, keep your hypoglycemia treatments or snacks handy. Like other breastfeeding mothers, you may find that you need to drink more sugar-free fluid than normal to prevent dehydration.

Sleeping

If you sleep when your baby sleeps, you will probably be "cat-napping" throughout the day. Unfortunately, this can result in hypoglycemia if you doze when you are due to eat a meal, or hyperglycemia if you sleep late and miss your injection time because you were awake most of the night. You may need to consider how to adapt your insulin regimen if an unpredictable sleeping pattern is causing serious swings in your blood glucose level.

Coping with stress

Looking after your new baby and trying to keep good control of your diabetes can be very stressful.

> **Q** **I'm really worried that I might have a hypoglycemic reaction when I'm alone with my baby. How can I make sure this doesn't happen?**
>
> **A** To guard against hypoglycemia, test your blood glucose level frequently. Keep glucose pills or glucose drinks in any room you might be using and if you feel a low blood glucose reaction coming on, treat it right away, even if you are unable to test your blood glucose level. Eat regularly, and have a snack if you get up to feed your baby at night. Don't nap or sleep on an empty stomach and try not to put your baby's feedings ahead of your own.

After working so hard to manage your blood glucose during pregnancy, it can be difficult to relax that very tight control and allow yourself to start aiming for good control again. You may even feel guilty if your blood glucose level is within the ideal range less often than it was when you were pregnant. Finding time to test, eat, and inject as you would like may also be a strain.

It is also very common for new mothers to feel low or miserable during the first few days or weeks after childbirth. Having diabetes won't make you any more or less likely to experience this mood change, known as the "baby blues," nor the more serious postpartum depression. However, feeling like this can affect your energy levels and your ability to manage your diabetes as well as your new baby's needs.

If you feel that you are not coping as well as you would like, you may find it helpful to talk to your health professional about different ways of dealing with motherhood and diabetes.

For everyday times when you are feeling low, simply talking to your health professional or family or friends can be helpful. Doing exercise when you can fit it in can be a useful way of relieving stress and meeting other people in a similar position to yourself. If you experience ongoing depression, you may need treatment (see pp.186–189). The more options you have for dealing with stressful times, the better you will be able to cope when they occur.

Myth OR TRUTH?

MYTH
You don't need to worry about your diabetes control once you've had your baby.

TRUTH
The tight control needed during pregnancy entails keeping your pre-meal blood glucose level below 5.3 mmol/L, and two hours after a meal below 6.7 mmol/L. After your baby is born, a blood glucose level higher than this, even for a day or two, is less likely to do harm, although your overall aim should still be to keep your level in the ideal range of 4–7 mmol/L. This will keep you well in the long term and reduce your risk of developing complications in the future.

Benefiting from health care

Having diabetes means that you probably use health care services more often than someone who doesn't have the condition. Regular health checkups are a routine part of your life, and you may need extra help if you are having difficulties with your diabetes management. Your health professional plays an important role in keeping you well, but the more knowledgeable you are about your diabetes and the more input you have, the better controlled your diabetes is likely to be.

Keeping yourself informed

To get the most from the health care you receive, you need to be informed about your own diabetes. The more you know about your condition, the more in control of your diabetes you can be. Your health professionals will help and support you, but you bear the greatest responsibility for your day-to-day diabetes care. Ask yourself the following questions to identify any gaps in your knowledge. If you are unsure of the facts, make a list of the questions you cannot answer so that you can ask them at your next appointment.

■ **WHAT TYPE OF DIABETES DO YOU HAVE?** This information is vital to enable you to understand your treatment and look after yourself properly. The type of diabetes you have always remains the same (unless you have gestational diabetes, see pp.144–145) even if

your treatment changes over time. For example, if you have type 2 diabetes and start insulin treatment, you still have type 2 diabetes.

■ **WHAT TARGETS ARE YOU AND YOUR HEALTH PROFESSIONAL AIMING FOR?** Targets given throughout this book are a general guide for everyone, but there may be specific A1C levels, home monitoring results, or blood pressure levels that you and your health professional want to achieve. If your diabetes has been out of control for a while, for example, it will probably take time to improve your levels and your targets might change from one appointment to the next. Knowing what your targets are will help you work with your health professional to achieve them.

■ **WHAT TREATMENT ARE YOU TAKING FOR YOUR DIABETES?** Knowing the names of your pills or insulin is helpful, particularly if you have appointments

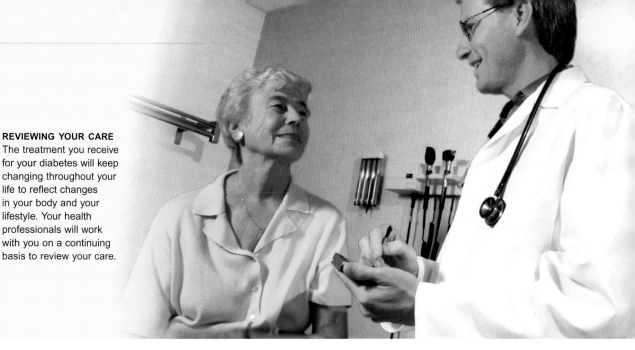

REVIEWING YOUR CARE
The treatment you receive for your diabetes will keep changing throughout your life to reflect changes in your body and your lifestyle. Your health professionals will work with you on a continuing basis to review your care.

with health professionals who do not know you very well. Part of your responsibility is to take your medication at the right times, such as in relation to meals, so that it is as effective as possible. It is also very important to take your treatment regularly, every day.

■ **ARE YOU DEVELOPING ANY LONG-TERM COMPLICATIONS OF DIABETES?** When you have your health checkups, you should be told what the results are.

> **Q** How often do I need to make an appointment to see my health professional—is it only four times a year?

> **A** Aside from your 3-monthly checkup, additional appointments depend on specific aspects of your diabetes care. For example, if any of your pills change, you will need to see your health professional soon to assess whether this has helped. More urgent problems, such as foot ulcers, may necessitate more frequent visits.

Therefore, you should know if there are any changes in your eyes, kidneys, feet, or heart, what changes to look for, and in what situations you should ask to be seen urgently.

■ **ARE THERE ANY OTHER HEALTH PROBLEMS CONNECTED TO YOUR DIABETES?**
Diabetes is a complex disease that can affect other aspects of your health (or vice versa). If you are unsure whether other health problems, for example stomach upsets or aches and pains, are related to your diabetes, you should clarify this at your next appointment, and make sure you understand the answers you are given.

Getting the most from your appointments

You will probably develop a regular relationship with one or two people, and see other health professionals occasionally. You may have all your health checkups performed by

Your health care professionals will help and support you, but you bear the greatest responsibility for your day-to-day diabetes care.

"The health professionals I have seen have given me helpful advice. They are always prepared to listen to my concerns and fears, however irrational these seem." SHELLEY

COMMENT It's very important to have open conversations with health professionals so that they can help you deal with your diabetes. If you don't voice your concerns, you may find it difficult to deal with them on your own. The expertise offered by your health professional can be invaluable—so don't hesitate to make the best use of it.

MONITORING YOUR HEALTH
During your annual checkup, your health professional will perform a number of tests, including checking your blood pressure, to assess your overall health.

different people or by one individual, depending on how services are organized in your area. Routine tests (such as having your eyes photographed or your feet examined) can be carried out by any health professional trained to perform that test. However, if you start to develop problems (with your eyes or feet, for example), you should expect to see someone who is specifically trained to treat and monitor those problems and provide you with more specific advice.

Preparing for your annual checkup

Your annual diabetes checkup is a two-way consultation between you and your health professional. Although you will have other appointments outside of the annual checkup, this yearly overview is an important part of your diabetes care. You have the opportunity to ask questions about your diabetes and discuss anything that is bothering you. Your health professional needs to know how you've been managing your diabetes so that he or she can assess whether any changes are necessary and help you with any concerns.

It's important to prepare for your appointment so that you can give your health professional as much information as possible and work together to decide on the best course of action. Before your appointment, write down any of the following:

- A regularly fluctuating blood glucose level.
- Side effects to medication.
- Changes you have made to your insulin or medication.
- Problems with equipment.
- Questions about new equipment or treatment.
- Lifestyle changes you have made or are planning, such as a new job or travel plans.

• If you are planning a pregnancy.
• Any difficulties with coping or keeping up your diabetes care.

During your annual checkup

As part of your annual checkup, your health professional will do the following or arrange for it to be done:
• Perform an A1C test to measure your long-term blood glucose level (see pp.66–67).
• Perform blood and urine tests to check kidney function and blood fat levels.
• Check your weight and body mass index (BMI).
• Examine your legs and feet to check your skin, circulation, and nerve supply.
• Check your blood pressure.
• Examine your eyes.
• Examine your injection sites if you are taking insulin.

If any problems are found, you will be referred for the appropriate treatment. You should feel free to talk about how you are coping with your diabetes at home, work, school, or college, and to raise any issues you might be concerned about, such as stress, physical activity, healthy eating, smoking or alcohol consumption, and sexual problems.

If at any time you don't understand what is being said, or you are unclear about any terms used, ask for an explanation. You can also discuss with your health professional the timing of your next appointment. You may wish to give yourself some time to try a new treatment or lifestyle change in order to see the benefits, or you may prefer to return to the clinic earlier if you feel you need some support in making any changes.

After your annual checkup

If you need to make any changes to your diabetes care, you should know why these changes need to be made, what effects they will have, and what to do if the changes do not produce the desired result. If you are asked to attend any other clinic appointment, make sure that you understand why it is necessary. It's a good idea to write down important information—after a long discussion you may not be able to remember everything that has been said.

To make sure that you leave your checkup with all the knowledge you need, make a note of the following:
• How your diabetes is and whether there are any concerns about your present or future health.
• Changes (if any) you need to make to your pills or insulin, including how often you take your medication and at what times of the day.
• What effect any change in treatment will have—how quickly it will work, how much it will affect your blood glucose level, what side effects you should look out for, and what action to take should they occur.
• Any additional treatment or appointments you need.
• Who to contact (and how) if you need help or advice before your next appointment.

Practical tips

CONTACTING YOUR HEALTH PROFESSIONAL

You should contact your health professional between appointments if you are experiencing any of the following:
• Frequent or severe low blood glucose levels.
• A consistently high blood glucose level.
• Injuries to your feet that are not healing.
• Sudden changes in your vision.
• Problems with medication or equipment.
• Feeling unable to cope.

If at any time you don't understand what is being said, or you are unclear about any terms used, ask for an explanation.

Children and teenagers

Diabetes can develop in babies or toddlers, later during childhood, during the teenage years, or beyond. Although age does not affect the type of treatment, diabetes care can be tailored to a child's needs at each stage of his or her development.

As a parent of a young child with diabetes, you bear the greatest responsibility for managing the condition. You need to inform caregivers; make sure your child is able to eat at the right time; monitor his or her blood glucose level and act on the results; inject insulin; and deal with low blood sugar.

As a parent of a school-aged child with diabetes, you need to communicate with teachers. Increasingly, your child will understand the importance of good blood glucose control and preventing hypoglycemic episodes, and you can work together to achieve this.

Teenagers and young adults are able to care more for their own diabetes with support from parents. Although teenagers may sometimes feel that diabetes restricts their independence, by becoming adept at integrating diabetes into their lifestyle, they can manage it successfully, and still live their life to the full.

Babies and young children

Caring for a baby or young child with diabetes places many demands on you as a parent. You need to give insulin injections, perform blood tests, and make sure that your child eats foods that have a beneficial effect on his or her diabetes. You also need to know how to act at times when your child is reluctant to let you do these things, what to do when his or her blood glucose level is too low, and how to care for your child when he or she is ill.

Myth OR TRUTH?

MYTH
Babies can't get diabetes.

TRUTH Although it is rare, babies of even a few months old have been diagnosed with type 1 diabetes. In fact, there is an increase in diabetes in children under the age of 5 in many countries.

Diabetes, your child, and you

It is rare for children under five to develop diabetes, but type 1 diabetes can occur in babies when they are only a few months old. Type 2 diabetes is just now being found in children under five. The symptoms of diabetes, such as urinating a lot and being very thirsty, are the same in children under five as in adults (see pp.18–19). Symptoms can become apparent very quickly—over a few days or a week—you might have noticed that your child's diaper needed changing more often, or that he or she started to wet the bed, or needed extra feedings and drinks.

Discovering that your young child has diabetes can give rise to many emotions: you may feel angry, upset, guilty, helpless, or anxious, and you may worry whether you will be able to cope with the level of care your

child will need every day. Because your child is so young, you will have the responsibility for looking after his or diabetes, which can make your job as a parent even more demanding. Your young child with diabetes needs food at regular intervals, blood tests, and insulin injections. Your child might not yet be able to tell you how he or she feels, so making sure that his or her blood glucose does not fall to a level at which hypoglycemia (see pp.102–109) can occur is also your responsibility.

However, you are not alone. You have the full support of diabetes health professionals as you learn more about diabetes and what you need to do to take care of your child.

It is important to take your child to regular diabetes visits and to talk with diabetes health professionals on a regular basis to discuss your child's growth and development, as well as

REGULAR EATING
Encouraging your child to eat regular meals and snacks containing complex carbohydrates is particularly important when he or she has diabetes.

his or her diabetes control. Keeping your child's blood glucose level between 4 and 7 millimoles per liter helps reduce the risk of complications when he or she is older.

Telling other people

Your family and friends will probably be concerned about your child's diabetes and they will almost certainly want to know more about it. In general, it's up to you to decide how much to say and to whom, but you will need to give more detailed information to people who care for your child, such as child care staff, babysitters, or caregivers.

When you tell people that your young child has diabetes, you will probably find that they respond in a variety of ways. People who are close to you may be upset and unsure how to treat your child. You may find it difficult to support and reassure others when it is all new to you, too,

but it is important to try to help people understand what you are going through and to appreciate how they are feeling too. If you have other children, they should also feel included in what is happening.

Whoever you talk to, you will probably find that everyone has something to say about diabetes, regardless of whether it is relevant to you and your child. When dealing with other people's reactions, you might want to prepare yourself with some stock answers to common

My experience

"Sometimes our daughter feels jealous of the attention her brother gets ... it hasn't been easy. When she tries to get involved with his diabetes it usually ends in fighting!" VICKY

COMMENT Siblings of children with diabetes can sometimes feel left out. They may start to behave differently in an effort to get more of your attention. If this happens, you may need to spend time alone with them so that they feel "special" too.

As your child grows, he or she will need to eat enough carbohydrate at mealtimes and throughout the day to keep his or her blood glucose level in the recommended range without going over it.

questions such as "What's diabetes?" "How did he or she get it?", or "Will he or she grow out of it?". If people try to give you advice, you could answer, "Thank you, I'll think about that," or "I've been told diabetes is very individual." You may sometimes receive conflicting advice from other people or health professionals—talk this through with your diabetes health professional to see how it relates specifically to your child's diabetes.

■ **TALKING TO CAREGIVERS** You need to make sure that anyone who looks after your child is given enough information about your child's diabetes, for example:
- What diabetes means.
- Your child's eating and drinking requirements.
- What treatments and blood glucose tests your child needs and when.
- Symptoms that might suggest hyperglycemia.
- Symptoms that might suggest hypoglycemia.
- What to do if your child has a hypoglycemic episode.
- What to do if your child is unwell.
- Your contact details at all times.
- Your physician's contact details.

Your child's caregiver will probably want to ask lots of questions and may be worried or even frightened about giving injections or testing your child's blood. Reassure him or her by demonstrating exactly what is involved. You may need to repeat the information often before it becomes familiar to your child's caregiver.

Eating and drinking

Your young child needs a variety of foods to make sure that he or she grows and develops healthily. If you are breastfeeding, feeding on demand will help fulfill your child's nutritional needs, although you may need to supplement breast milk with bottle feeding at times when your baby's blood glucose is low. If low blood glucose is a constant problem, reducing your child's insulin dose will be helpful.

As you introduce your child to more foods, you will need to include those with complex carbohydrate, such as bread, pasta, and potatoes. As your child grows, he or she will need to eat enough carbohydrate at meals and throughout the day to keep his or her blood glucose level in the recommended range but not over it (see p.157). Snacks between meals could include fruit juice or milkshakes, cereal bars, or fruit.

Your child may be fussy about food at times and his or her eating pattern may vary a lot. This can be frustrating when you want to encourage your child to eat in order to prevent him or her from having hypoglycemia.

If your child refuses food, keep calm. Have an alternative prepared, perhaps a meal or snack that you know your child particularly likes, that will tempt him or her to eat. Be careful not to offer more than one or two choices though: if your child learns that he or she can command many more options, your mealtimes could become a battleground.

You won't do your child any harm if some meals are higher in fat or sugar than others. It is the overall content of his or her food intake that matters. For example, you can compensate for a lunch of fish sticks and fries by giving your child fruit as a snack later, or a salad or chopped vegetables and a baked potato.

Bedtime snacks

You need to make sure that your child has eaten enough of an evening meal to keep his or her blood glucose from falling overnight, especially if he or she usually sleeps through until morning. If you don't think your child has had enough food and you can't fit in a snack before bedtime, you may need to test your child's blood glucose later in the evening in case he or she becomes hypoglycemic. If necessary, give your child a drink or easy-to-eat snack. If low blood glucose becomes a regular event, you may need to reduce your child's insulin dose at the evening mealtime. As your child grows older and the time between his or her evening meal and bedtime gets longer, you can start a routine of a snack before he or she goes to bed. Bars containing cornstarch help keep the blood glucose level up.

Eating out

There is no reason why you shouldn't eat out when your child has diabetes, whether at a restaurant or a friend's house.

Fast food, takeout, and party food are all okay, even if they may contain too much fat, salt, and sugar to be good for your child on a regular basis. They just shouldn't be eaten every day or every week. If you are not sure what will be available, pack an emergency supply of foods your child will eat (in addition to glucose and longer-acting, carbohydrate-containing food to treat hypoglycemia).

Blood glucose control

Keeping good control of your child's blood glucose level is essential right from the start: what you do now can make a difference to his or her health as an adult and reduce the risk of long-term complications such as eye, kidney, and nerve problems. Good blood glucose control is also important for healthy growth in young children—a high blood glucose level can reduce the effect of growth hormones. Good control for young children is the same as for anyone else with diabetes: the target is for A1C levels to be 7 percent or below (see p.66) and blood glucose targets geared to the child's age.

You won't always be able to achieve results in this range, but by keeping

(see p.66)

Practical tips

SUPERVISING YOUR CHILD'S FOOD INTAKE

- Mealtimes are important for social as well as for nutritional reasons—don't make them a carbohydrate battleground! All young children will eat when they are hungry.
- Don't worry if your child's diet is not 100% healthy— it's the overall balance that matters.
- If you're having problems, ask your health professional about ways of matching your child's insulin to his or her current eating pattern.

FAST FOODS
Most children enjoy fries, which, although high in fat, won't do any harm if eaten every so often. If you cook fries at home, you can reduce fat by choosing oven-baked varieties.

TRUTH?

MYTH
You don't have to worry about good diabetes control until your child gets older.

TRUTH
However young your child is when he or she develops diabetes, good control is essential from the start and is associated with better health in later life. Children are not protected from the effects of poor blood glucose control even though complications might not show until they are adults.

records of your child's blood glucose test results, you will probably become expert at identifying patterns of highs or lows and working out what to do about them. Taking action as soon as you notice a pattern of blood glucose levels outside the recommended range will limit the effect.

Testing your child's blood glucose level and giving insulin injections may be hard for you, especially at first, but these tasks are essential. To attain the best diabetes control possible, you will need to test your child's blood glucose regularly before and/or after meals and whenever your child engages in a new or unusual activity. You can then adjust your child's treatment, activity, or food intake according to the results.

Identifying patterns

Any changes you make to your child's treatment, activity, or food intake should be based on a pattern of results rather than an individual test result. For example, if your child has a blood glucose reading of more than 10 millimoles per liter at lunchtime

for three consecutive days, this is a pattern for which you should try to find a cause. Ask yourself questions, such as "Is he or she eating or drinking anything different at the moment?", "Has he or she been less active than usual?", or "Is he or she sick?". Once you identify the cause, you can take action—for the situation described above, you might change what your child is eating for breakfast. If you can't find an obvious reason for high readings, your child may simply need more insulin to match his or her growth—an increase in his or her morning dose is probably necessary for this situation.

Follow up any action with a test to find out whether or not a change has worked. (For more information on making adjustments, see pp.90–95.)

Even if your child has a slightly high blood glucose level and seems well, don't allow this to continue for more than a few days. A higher than normal blood glucose level for longer than this could increase the chance of your child feeling sick or being at risk of long-term complications when he or she is older.

Good diabetes control also entails avoiding low readings that could lead to hypoglycemia (see pp.102–109). It is certain to happen occasionally, but serious or long-lasting episodes can be frightening for you both. You can prevent these by keeping your child's blood glucose above 4 millimoles per liter.

There will be periods when it is very difficult to keep your child's

My experience

"Our 8-year-old has had diabetes since he was 4. We have tried most types of insulin—from one injection a day to multiple doses, from half a unit at a time to several units. It's trial and error. You need patience and perseverance." IAIN

COMMENT The insulin requirements of a growing child change constantly. You will need to try different insulins and regimens from time to time to find one that best suits your child at a particular stage of development.

blood glucose level within the ideal range, particularly as your child grows older, bigger, and takes part in new activities. Sometimes your child might need a change of insulin type or regimen (see pp.87–95). Discuss the options with your health professional. You can be sure that more changes will be needed before too long!

Tests and injections

Although you might find it difficult to inject your child every day, he or she needs insulin to live, and blood glucose tests will always be part of his or her everyday life. The exact times you test and give insulin each day will vary but will follow a general pattern. For example, your child will need an insulin injection around one or more of his or her mealtimes and blood glucose tests either just before or two hours after meals.

The doses of insulin will also vary. For up to two years after diagnosis, your child may experience a "honeymoon period," when he or she is likely to need only very small doses of insulin. Once this period is over, your child will need more insulin. You may also need to increase the insulin dose when your child has a growth spurt. Learning to adjust your child's insulin is part of learning to live with diabetes, and your health professional will help you with this.

Coping with tantrums

There will be times when your child is not willing to have an injection or to have his or her blood glucose

tested. Think about how you encourage your child to take care of other aspects of his or her health, such as bathing or toothbrushing, and try to incorporate diabetes care into his or her routine in the same way. Bear in mind that very young children may fiercely resist having an injection or test, but are easily distracted immediately afterward.

Even if you sometimes feel guilty about giving your child an injection or doing a blood test when he or she is upset, be careful about the kind of reward you give afterward. Having a cuddle, reading a book, or playing with a favorite toy together can help your child link injection or test time with a pleasurable experience, but rewards such as new activities, new toys, or even food can be difficult to deliver every day.

Doing a blood test on yourself or inserting one of your child's clean needles into your skin when you are alone may help you understand what testing and injecting feels like in reality.

Dealing with hypoglycemia

Hypoglycemic episodes are a side effect of insulin treatment so your child will have them from time to time, especially if you are keeping good control of his or her diabetes. If your child is too young to talk, the symptoms of hypoglycemia will be difficult to recognize at first and you will need to be alert for signs that come on quickly, such as becoming very uncoordinated, sweaty, pale,

Practical tips

TESTING OR INJECTING A RELUCTANT CHILD

- Explain what you are going to do and do it immediately. Don't say that you'll do something "in 5 minutes"—this will increase any sense of anxiety.
- Hold your child firmly and securely on your knee as you test or inject.
- Ask other family members to help if necessary.
- Allow your child to help if he or she wants to (and is old enough).
- Cuddle and praise your child when the test or injection is finished.
- Afterward, quickly get back to what the two of you were doing beforehand.

TREATING A SEVERE HYPOGLYCEMIC EPISODE

If a severe hypoglycemic episode is untreated, there is a risk that your child could become unconscious or have a seizure. A seizure doesn't mean that your child has epilepsy; it is the brain's reaction to insufficient glucose. You will need to keep calm and take the following measures to help your child recover.

1 If your child is having a seizure, make sure his mouth is clear to breathe. If you are still worried, call an ambulance.

2 If your child can breathe normally, lay him on his side or hold him with his head tilted back slightly to keep his airway clear.

3 Prepare, or ask someone else to prepare, a glucagon injection (see p.109) and give it to your child in his arm, buttock, or leg. Don't try to give him anything to eat or drink.

4 When your child has regained consciousness, he might vomit as a result of the glucagon injection. Sit him up and check his blood glucose level as soon as it is practical to do so.

5 Once he is more alert, give him some food or drink that contains carbohydrate to keep his blood glucose level raised.

6 Check his blood glucose level every half hour until it is above 4 millimoles per liter and stay with him until you are both feeling better.

silent, or staring into space. Your child's warning signs are individual but tend to be the same each time, so it's important to learn what they are. You also need to be aware that your child could have a severe hypoglycemic episode if he or she:
- Has been very physically active but hasn't had less insulin or more food to compensate.
- Eats less than usual over several meals.
- Has had too much insulin.
- Becomes overheated, for example, in hot weather.
- Has a vomiting illness.

A blood glucose test will confirm whether your child's blood glucose level has fallen below 4 millimoles per liter, which means that he or she is hypoglycemic.

If you can't do a test, and you think your child is hypoglycemic because of his or her symptoms, it won't do any harm to give your baby a breastfeeding or bottle feeding, or your young child glucose tablets, a glucose drink, or glucose gel (see p.106) to raise his or her blood glucose level. The sooner you treat it, the sooner your child will recover.

Since hypoglycemia can be unpredictable, it's useful to keep glucose tablets or a sugary drink available to treat them. You can also limit the risk by giving your child a carbohydrate snack at bedtime or waking him or her for a feeding or snack during the night. During the day, regular feeds or meals and snacks will help balance insulin doses. If your child eats much less than usual at a mealtime or over several mealtimes, you may need to reduce his or her next dose of insulin.

If you know that your child will be particularly active, such as at a party, or running around outside, you can give him or her more to eat or a reduced insulin dose beforehand. Extra activity at any time can cause your child's blood glucose level to fall several hours later. To avoid serious hypoglycemia as a result, especially at night, give your child extra food over a few hours after his or her activity.

Coping with illness

From time to time, your child, like any other, will become sick. Children are not more likely to be ill just because they have diabetes, but if their diabetes is not well controlled and they have a high blood glucose level over an extended period of time, they may be more prone to infections. This is because glucose-rich blood provides an ideal environment in which germs can multiply.

When your child has diabetes, any illness can affect his or her blood glucose level and vice versa. Children's blood glucose can either rise or fall, so their doses of insulin may need to be increased or decreased. The golden rule is to continue giving your child his or her insulin every day and not to stop for any reason, to prevent diabetic ketoacidosis (see p.113). Even if your child is not eating, he or she must continue to have insulin, although you may need to give very small doses. Doing more blood glucose tests when your child is unwell will help you decide how much insulin to give. Discussing how to deal with illness with your health professional and having information about what to do will help you cope when your child becomes sick.

To care for your sick child, give sugar-free drinks to keep him or her hydrated and test his or her blood glucose level at least four times a day. If your child has a high temperature, remove most of his or her clothing, and use a washcloth moistened with tepid water to cool his or her skin. Your child should also have plenty of cool drinks and may need a temperature-lowering medicine from your health professional or pharmacy.

Young children can become sick quickly, which can make their blood glucose level difficult to control. If you can't bring your child's blood glucose under control while he or she is ill, contact your health professional for advice.

If your child is vomiting and cannot keep any food or drink down at all, take him or her to a hospital emergency room immediately or call an ambulance. In this situation, your child will need insulin and fluid via an infusion to prevent him or her from becoming seriously ill with diabetic ketoacidosis (see p.113).

If your child is vomiting and cannot keep any food or drink down at all, take him or her to a hospital emergency room immediately or call an ambulance.

School-age children

Whether your child has recently been diagnosed with diabetes or has had diabetes from a young age, his or her school years present new challenges. As your child grows and becomes more independent, it is important to encourage his or her involvement in diabetes care, with initial supervision of injections and testing. You also need to develop a system of diabetes care that fits in with a school routine; obtaining the support of school staff will help keep your child's diabetes well controlled.

A child with diabetes can do everything any other child can do, but blood glucose control is important to keep him or her healthy.

Diabetes, your child, and you

Children between the ages of 5 and 12 who develop diabetes are most likely to have type 1 diabetes, but more and more cases of type 2 diabetes in school-age children are being found. The symptoms of diabetes, including frequent urination, thirst, and weight loss, are the same in school-age children as in adults (see pp.18–19). You might notice that your child starts to wet the bed, is always drinking, and is much more tired than usual.

A school-age child with diabetes needs insulin injections or pills, blood tests, and a balanced food intake that includes plenty of carbohydrate foods. A child with diabetes can do everything that any other child can do, but good blood glucose control is important to keep him or her healthy now and to prevent complications associated with diabetes in the future. Good blood glucose control is also important to ensure your child's healthy physical development, since a consistently high blood glucose level can reduce the effectiveness of growth hormone.

As soon as your child starts school, he or she will be more independent, will be asking lots of questions, and making new friends. Your child is also likely to be very active; for example, going out more to other people's houses, and enjoying school trips and parties. As a parent, it's important to balance caring for your child's diabetes with allowing him or her to simply get on with the social aspects of growing up. You can also help your child on the path to self-sufficiency by encouraging his or her involvement in diabetes care. Until your child is older, you will be the best judge of what he or she is

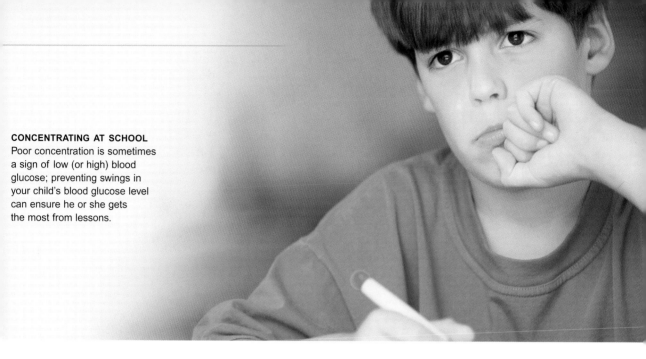

CONCENTRATING AT SCHOOL
Poor concentration is sometimes
a sign of low (or high) blood
glucose; preventing swings in
your child's blood glucose level
can ensure he or she gets
the most from lessons.

capable of and when. Sometimes
your child will want to be involved in
his or her diabetes care and sometimes
he or she won't. This is normal, and
adapting to it is part of being a parent.

If your child has recently been
diagnosed with diabetes, you will
have many different feelings, worries,
and questions. You may feel shocked
at first, and possibly overwhelmed.
You will have the opportunity of
discussing the way you feel with a
health professional. You may also find
it very helpful to get together and
share experiences, successes, and
worries with other parents of children
with diabetes.

Telling other people

How many people you tell and how
much information you provide about
your child's diabetes is a personal
decision and depends to a large
extent on how involved other people
are in caring for your child's diabetes.

■ **TALKING TO TEACHERS** Your child's
teachers may know little about
diabetes, and, consequently, you may
wish to arrange a meeting with them
in order to explain your child's
needs. Your health professional can
accompany you to the meeting
to advise school staff about diabetes
and address their concerns. The

Q **My daughter has had diabetes
for six months and has gradually
needed less and less insulin. Will she
stop needing it altogether?**

A It sounds as though your
daughter is experiencing what is
called the "honeymoon period," which
can last anything up to 2 years after
type 1 diabetes is diagnosed. During
this time, the pancreas seems to
recover a little and starts producing
insulin again, so only small doses of
injected insulin are needed. However,
at some stage within 2 years, your
daughter's insulin-producing cells will
stop working altogether and she will
require larger doses of insulin again.

MANAGING YOUR CHILD'S INSULIN

• Make sure that your child hasn't had so many snacks or drinks that he or she can't eat at mealtimes. If you're worried about hypoglycemic reactions between meals or at school, you may need to reduce your child's insulin doses rather than overdo the snacks.

• If you can't predict how much or when your child will eat, you may wish to use an insulin that you can give up to 15 minutes after a meal. Ask your health professional for advice.

• It's the overall control of your child's diabetes that matters, not a single blood glucose result. These won't be perfect all the time—no one's are!

more information and clear instructions you can provide, the more confident teachers and staff are likely to feel about their ability to care for your child if he or she experiences a hypoglycemic episode at school.

One way to communicate with teachers about your child's diabetes is to use a notebook. You and your child's teacher can write in the book to keep in touch and share relevant information. For example, you might want to tell the teacher that your child's blood glucose level is high that day; or the teacher might notice that your child needs to go to the bathroom more often.

Your child may have a hypoglycemic episode at school if he or she is not able to have a meal or snack at the usual time, has not had enough to eat, or has used up more energy than normal, such as during an extra gym class or a particularly energetic game at recess. You will need to warn the school staff that a hypoglycemic reaction might occur immediately or an hour or two later, and that your child will need to take or be given glucose—in the form of pills or a drink—quickly. Your child should keep emergency supplies to treat a hypoglycemic attack with him or her at all times. You should also tell school staff what they should do if your child becomes unconscious as a result of hypoglycemia (see pp.102–109).

Target blood glucose ranges vary and depend on a child's age and other factors. Talk with your child's doctor to determine the target range that's best for him or her. If you are worried about hypoglycemic reactions occurring at school, or they are happening often, your child may need a different insulin regimen. Talk to your health professional about the choices available.

Eating and drinking

The principles of healthy eating (see pp.30–43) are the same for a child with diabetes as for any other child—his or her meals should be based on complex carbohydrates with some protein, and fat, sugar, and salt in moderation. Also, encourage your child to eat several portions of fruit and vegetables a day.

In general, your child needs three meals a day, plus three snacks—one in the morning, one in the afternoon, and one at bedtime. Snacks between meals will boost your child's energy and balance with his or her insulin to prevent hypoglycemia. However, because your child's appetite will vary, you'll have to be flexible about how much he or she eats.

On some days, for example, you may need to give your child an extra snack to compensate for an unusually small lunch. On other days, he or she might be particularly hungry at dinner time and ask for extra helpings. Learning to adjust your child's insulin dose to accommodate new eating patterns can be very helpful.

If your child is going to be especially active, on a school sports day, for example, he or she will need an extra carb-containing snack beforehand and may need extra food several hours later (see p.169).

Eating at school

There is no reason why your child shouldn't have school meals. School menus are usually based on healthy eating guidelines, so your child should be offered a variety of good foods.

If your child is not willing or able to eat enough carbohydrate at lunchtime, you may need to ask teachers and staff if it is possible to offer alternative foods. You should also discuss whether your child may need to be among the first to be served at lunchtime, or be in the same sitting every day, in order to prevent a hypoglycemic episode.

Your child will need a snack mid-morning and at afternoon break to balance his or her morning insulin. There may be times when your child needs to eat a snack earlier, such as if he or she feels hypoglycemic or recess is delayed. Make sure that school staff are aware of this and will allow your child to eat a snack when necessary. Small, easy-to-eat snacks are especially useful at these times.

You might prefer to give your child packed lunches, so that you can choose healthy foods that he or she likes. Your child can also play a part in choosing and making packed lunches. You could include any of the following foods in a packed lunch or as snacks.

- Bread, such as bagels or sandwiches with low-fat fillings, rice cakes, or breadsticks.
- Low-fat potato chips or small cheese crackers.
- Fruit—dried, canned in natural juice, or fresh—in small easy-to-eat pieces, if necessary.
- Individual packs of cereal with lowfat milk.
- Cereal bars.
- Fruit yogurt.
- Milkshake made with lowfat milk and fresh fruit or fruit yogurt.
- Two or three plain cookies, such as ginger snaps, or crackers.

Whether your child has school meals or packed lunches, knowing the answers to the following questions will help you plan his or her food intake throughout the school day:
- What time does the school day start and finish?
- Are children allowed to eat at morning and afternoon recess, and how often is recess delayed?

You might prefer to give your child packed lunches, so that you can choose healthy foods that he or she likes.

EATING AT LUNCHTIME
It's important to make sure that your child eats enough carbohydrate-containing foods at lunchtime to prevent hypoglycemia later in the day.

Alert your child's teacher to the possibility that a hypoglycemic reaction could occur on a school trip, and be sure that your child will be allowed to eat if necessary.

PARTY FOOD
No child wants to miss out on treats such as birthday cake, and there are ways to prevent or decrease the likelihood of a resulting high blood glucose level.

• What time is lunch; is it different for children who have school meals than those who have brought a packed lunch?

• When does your child have a gym class, and how often do unplanned physical activities take place?

Eating at friends' houses

Your child may be invited to other children's houses for meals or parties. Because these are not everyday events, you can help your child enjoy high-fat or sugary snacks and cakes, and keep his or her blood glucose from rising too high. If you are concerned that your child's blood glucose will rise too much, you could ask the person in charge to have sugar-free drinks available or provide them yourself.

If your child tends to rush around with friends playing party games, for example, the energy he or she uses will balance out any extra food he or she has eaten. If your child is quieter and less active, however, he or she

may need a little extra insulin that day. Sometimes the excitement of his or her own birthday parties even causes the guest of honor's blood glucose to go low!

School trips

On school trips, when meals might be earlier or later than usual, your child will need a few extra snacks and hypoglycemia supplies in case of delays. Be sure to pack plenty of snacks. On these occasions, it will not do your child any harm to eat more than usual even if it causes his or her blood glucose to rise for that day.

Alert your child's teacher to the possibility that a hypoglycemic reaction could occur on a school trip, and make sure that your child will be allowed to eat a snack if necessary. Remind the person in charge that your child's blood glucose level might rise as a result of excitement, so he or she may need to go to the bathroom more often or be particularly thirsty (see Hyperglycemia, pp.110–113). Before the school trip, make sure that you have the following information:

• Leaving and returning times and whether these are likely to be delayed.

• Arrangements for snacks and meals during the trip.

• Name of the person in charge—is it the usual teacher or someone else?

• Arrangements for contacting parents if there should be a problem.

• Arranging for checking blood glucose and taking injections—will your child be responsible for these, or will the person in charge do them?

Blood glucose control

Good control of your child's diabetes is meeting the target blood glucose range most of the time and an A1C level (see p.66) of approximately 7 percent. The more often you achieve your goal levels, the greater the chances of preventing long-term complications in adulthood. You'll need to test your child's blood glucose level regularly and adjust his or her treatment, activity, or food intake according to the results. Identifying and treating patterns is more useful than acting on an individual result (see pp.62–75).

Changing routines, activity levels, and growing rates all affect blood glucose and insulin needs, and, as a result, your child's blood glucose readings won't always be within the ideal range. You will need to work closely with your doctor and diabetes

educator in order to make the adjustments that your growing child will need. You and your child must also work together to note changes in everything from his or her stress levels to diabetes symptoms so that you can report them to your doctor or diabetes specialist and correlate them with increases or decreases in your child's blood glucose level.

Children can become enthusiastic about aiming for normal readings if they know they will feel better. Test and adjust insulin or food to achieve a normal blood glucose level until your child feels well at these levels (see pp.90–95 for more information on adjusting doses).

Tests and injections

Your child will need to have tests and injections every day in order to keep his or her diabetes under good control. To help your child learn that caring for his or her diabetes is an important part of the daily routine, it's a good idea to treat tests and injections like any other health-related activity, such as hand-washing or tooth-brushing.

Practical tips

INVOLVING CHILDREN IN DIABETES CARE

• Explain simply and clearly to your child what insulin is for and why he or she needs to learn how to test and inject, so that it becomes a familiar story.

• If your child needs a break with tests or injections, take over for a few days. Children like to be independent, so they will take charge again eventually!

• To maintain or refresh your child's interest in his or her diabetes, look at a new insulin devices or blood glucose meters with your diabetes educator—there are types available to suit all tastes.

• Make sure that your child carries a supply of glucose and some form of medical identification at all times.

My experience

"I took care of my diabetes from the age of 11. I tried many insulins to see what suited me best and lots of blood glucose meters to find which gave me the quickest results." SHELLEY

COMMENT Some children are able to manage their own diabetes from an early age and make decisions about what's important to them, such as how to make it easier to do tests or injections. There is a wide range of equipment that is easy to use and appealing to children.

PREVENTING PROBLEMS

● Keep a record of your child's daily blood glucose results, so you can identify patterns and decide whether anything needs to change.

● Injecting constantly in the same site causes lumps and insulin isn't absorbed properly when injected in lumpy skin. Change your child's injection site regularly and teach him or her to do this himself or herself.

INJECTION TIMES
Sometimes children are happy to take responsibility for their own injections; at other times they may lose all interest in looking after their diabetes and you will need to take charge for a little while.

There is no ideal age for your child to start doing his or her own blood tests and injections. He or she may want to start doing it in elementary school or may not show an interest until high school. Your child might be more ready to do one or the other first, or need your help at some times more than others. You can help most by going along with what your child feels able to do, and making sure that tests and injections are performed with as little fuss as possible, whoever does them.

Involving children as much as possible in working out what their test results mean and what changes you need to make to their insulin dose, food intake, or activity levels will help them toward taking responsibility for their own diabetes. Praise your child for looking after his or her diabetes well, but avoid allowing him or her to negotiate testing or injection times too much, as this can easily create a frustrating daily battle.

Occasionally, you or your child will need to change the type or timing of his or her insulin and the frequency of tests, perhaps because your child is having a growth spurt, eating more or less of certain foods, has a different routine at school, or has started to socialize more outside your home. Ask your health professional to help you choose the best system from the wide range of insulins, injection devices, and blood glucose meters available.

Dealing with hypoglycemia

Trying to keep good control of your child's diabetes will inevitably lead to occasional hypoglycemic episodes. Your doctor will discuss with you the levels at which it is a particular risk. The signs of hypoglycemia are usually similar each time, so you, your child, and teachers can learn to recognize them.

The older your child, the more able he or she will be to take action or tell someone when symptoms occur. Your child should carry glucose at all times and, if he or she is able to recognize the warning signs of a hypoglycemia, should learn to take glucose before a reaction becomes severe. Sometimes, however, your child will be unaware of the signs or won't tell you how he or she feels. Both you and your child's teachers

Q What happens if my daughter has a hypoglycemic episode in the night that I don't know about?

A Her liver will react to the hypoglycemia, by converting stored glycogen into glucose and releasing it into her bloodstream. As a result, your daughter's blood glucose level could be high in the morning, and she may also have a headache and feel tired. You might check her blood glucose at 3 am for several nights to see if she is going too low. You can prevent hypoglycemia at night by giving your child extra food or less insulin in the evening.

need to be alert for sudden changes in behavior, such as your child being particularly naughty, argumentative, aggressive, or very sleepy. A blood test will confirm hypoglycemia but if you can't test, you won't do any harm by treating what seems to be a hypoglycemic attack right away (see pp.106–108).

Hypoglycemic reactions can also occur some time after your child has been physically active because his or her injected insulin will continue to work after the glucose in his or her body has been used for energy. However, it is important that your child is active because exercise helps keep his or her heart healthy, maintains a healthy body weight, and keeps blood pressure and cholesterol, levels within the recommended ranges. So if you are concerned about hypoglycemia, try changing the time of your child's insulin injection or reducing the dose before activity. If the activity is unplanned, give your child an extra carbohydrate snack. If the activity lasts longer than an hour, your child may need extra glucose in the form of a drink or pill during the activity, too.

Although you will want to protect your child against hypoglycemia, avoid the temptation to keep blood glucose consistently too high (above 10 millimoles per liter) in an effort to prevent these reactions. There is no guarantee that such measures will work because insulin levels in the bloodstream and the amount of energy used up by your child

> **My experience**
>
> *"It has been helpful to have a very good multidisciplinary pediatric diabetes team at the other end of the phone for help and advice. The team knows us as a family and that's great."* IAIN
>
> **COMMENT** Caring for a child with diabetes can sometimes be a challenge for the whole family, so it is reassuring to be able to contact health professionals who know you and your child and understand your situation.

throughout the day may vary a lot. In addition, a high blood glucose level can cause symptoms as well as putting your child at risk of health complications in the future.

Life at school

Your child's diabetes will not affect his or her ability to take part in school activities. Provided he or she is allowed to eat meals and snacks when necessary and you can plan for food needs, testing, and injections, school life shouldn't present any major obstacles.

Depending on your child's age, he or she may be able to do blood tests and injections during the school day. You and your health professional must write out a detailed plan for the school staff of the care your child needs daily, including snacks, and who is responsible for each task.

If school staff are worried about your child's diabetes, they may be unwilling to allow him or her to participate in some activities. If you believe that this is the case, talk to the principal and ask your health professional to help work out a solution.

Your child should carry glucose at all times and, if he or she is able to recognize the warning signs of hypoglycemia, should learn to take glucose before a hypoglycemic episode becomes severe.

Teenagers and young adults

This is the time when most childhood diabetes begins. Adolescence is a time of change; a teenager with diabetes has to deal not only with peer pressures, exams, and the effects of hormones but also with blood glucose control. As a parent, you need to be supportive. As a teenager, you need to cope with your feelings, eat and drink healthily when you can, and look after your diabetes in ways that suit your lifestyle. You also need to know how smoking, alcohol, and drugs can affect your diabetes.

Diabetes, your teenager, and you

Teenagers and young adults who develop diabetes are likely to have type 1 diabetes, previously known as juvenile onset diabetes. However, type 2 diabetes, which usually affects older people, is now being found in children and teenagers, too. Although only a few teenagers have been diagnosed with type 2 diabetes in the UK, in Canada, the numbers are higher, and rising rapidly. The rise in type 2 diabetes among the young is believed to be linked to sedentary lifestyles, increasing levels of obesity, and is seen more often in vulnerable populations. Many of the young people with type 2 diabetes are overweight at the time of diagnosis. If your teenager has developed type 2 diabetes or MODY (a form of diabetes similar to type 2; see p.16), it will need to be managed similarly to type 2 diabetes in an older person.

The symptoms of diabetes, including frequent urination, thirst, and weight loss, are the same in teenagers as in adults (see pp.18–19). Symptoms can come on very quickly —over a few days or a week—and you might notice that your teenager is more tired than usual and getting up at night to go to the bathroom or have a drink.

A teenager with type 1 diabetes needs insulin injections, blood tests, and a balanced food intake that

---

My experience

"I thought I must have done something wrong. I felt upset and confused ... I was worried about my mom since she was frightened, too. Then I met other people who were going through the same thing and I didn't feel quite so alone." JANE

COMMENT The feelings you have when you are first diagnosed with diabetes as a teenager can be very negative. It's reassuring to know that you aren't the only one and to talk to teenagers in the same position.

DEALING WITH DIABETES
It can be difficult to deal with your diabetes when you are a teenager or young adult. Taking time out to come to terms with your feelings and developing a strategy for fitting diabetes care into your busy life can help you feel more positive.

includes plenty of carbohydrate foods. Type 2 diabetes or MODY may be treated with healthy eating and physical activity, followed by pills and insulin injections when necessary. Whatever type of diabetes your teenager has, good diabetes care now is important to keep your teenager in the best of health and to prevent complications associated with diabetes in the future.

Whether your teenager has recently been diagnosed with diabetes or has had diabetes from a young age, the teenage years bring new challenges and pressures. The transition into adulthood is a time of physical and emotional change and growth, and the effects of hormones can be great. Relationships with peers can also be difficult at this time and the added pressure of exams or work may not help. Having diabetes can complicate your teenager's life even further and concern you as a parent, but there

are ways of working together to make the process of growing up as trouble-free as possible.

Out of concern and love, you may be tempted to try to keep control of your teenager's diabetes, but this is virtually impossible. It is your teenager's diabetes, and he or she must eventually take full responsibility for it. Try to develop a supportive rather than a controlling role.

Teenagers still need, and will respond to, rules and boundaries, even though they might argue about them endlessly. Be firm and consistent and treat diabetes care as you would any other aspect of your teenager's life that requires rules, such as coming home at a certain time or keeping his or her bedroom tidy. For example, you might insist that your teenager performs a minimum number of blood tests per day or per week; that he or she does not go out until he or she has taken

> Good diabetes care now is important to keep your teenager in the best of health and to prevent complications associated with diabetes in the future.

insulin and eaten; that he or she eats high-fat or high-sugar foods only occasionally; or that he or she attends doctor's appointments without argument. The more you involve teenagers in making decisions about what they are going to do, the more likely it is that they will stick to what has been agreed.

No parent is perfect and your relationship with your teenager and his or her diabetes will not always go smoothly. However, a teenager who is doing most or even some things that are important in looking after his or her diabetes deserves praise and encouragement. If you are worried that your teenager is not doing enough and none of your ideas seem to work, you will need help from

family, friends, or your health professional. When your teenager doesn't seem to listen to you, he or she will often be more receptive to friends, so ask for the support of anyone you think will encourage your teenager to keep on top of his or her diabetes management. You can also contact health professionals who work with teenagers.

As a parent, you want your child to grow up healthy and happy, and able to make his or her way in the world. On the other hand, your child probably wants to live for the moment and be one of the crowd. He or she may rebel against authority, experiment with activities, and test out different relationships. How teenagers treat their diabetes varies,

TALKING TO TEENAGERS
Good communication involves listening as well as talking, so it's important to give your teenager a fair hearing, even if you don't necessarily agree with what's being said.

but it is likely to be similar to the way in which they treat other aspects of their lives. They may realize the importance of the day-to-day tasks of caring for their diabetes, and fit them in without too much effort. On the other hand, they may see diabetes as setting them apart from their friends and try to make it less obvious by ignoring it or doing little in the way of testing or eating a healthy diet.

At the same time, your teenager's diabetes will be changing. The effect of hormones is likely to increase the amount of insulin he or she needs throughout adolescence. In addition, the pressures of taking exams or starting work, developing sexually, and possibly experimenting with alcohol or drugs will all affect his or her blood glucose level. So home blood tests and contact with your health professional continue to be important.

Talking to your teenager

Communication with your teenager may be straightforward and open or may sometimes consist of one-word answers, arguments, or even shouting matches or battles of will. In general, any talking is good, but the calmer, the better. Even if your teenager seems to reject your every word, the lines of communication must remain open for when he or she is ready to talk. There is no reason why you shouldn't let your teenager know what you think and feel about his or her diabetes, although it may help choose a time when you feel your child is at his or her most receptive.

Your feelings as a teenager

When you have diabetes it seems as though there is a lot to do to look after yourself. It can seem to get in the way of your day-to-day life and you won't always want to do your blood tests and injections, or think about when and what you're going to eat. The good news is that you are normal—no one, whether they have diabetes or not, can always do everything they are meant to in relation to their health.

The not-so-good news is that if you regularly don't take care of your diabetes you are very likely to be storing up problems for later on. You probably think that developing problems in 20 years' time sounds a long way off, but even then you will still be under 40 and you'll need your eyesight, healthy feet, and kidneys, and a strong heart for the rest of your life. You don't have to be perfect all the time to make sure this is the case for you, but you do need to work at it some of the time.

If you've just been diagnosed

You should be feeling a lot better now that you are taking insulin, and learning a lot of new information. Your health professional will be in touch with you regularly and you may feel ready to do all your tests and injections and eat the right things. Your friends and family will be paying a lot of attention to you at

---

Practical tips

KEEPING IN TOUCH WITH YOUR TEENAGER

- Learn how to say "yes" as well as "no."
- Don't ask too many questions about his or her diabetes—it may feel as though you are nagging.
- Listen calmly to anything he or she says.
- Let your teenager know that you respect, love, and support him or her.
- Try not to be too overprotective—allow your teenager to do what his or her friends do.
- Help your teenager work out his or her diabetes control and treatment for every type of situation.
- Encourage your teenager to come up with his or her own solutions to problems with diabetes control—he or she will learn more by experimenting than by simply following instructions.

the moment, partly out of concern for you and partly because it's all new to them, too. You will find that, as you get used to having diabetes, the novelty will wear off and you might become a bit bored or fed up with testing and injections, especially if you are feeling healthy again. However, it's important for you to try to find ways to keep going with your diabetes care.

If you've had diabetes for a while

Diabetes sometimes gets in the way of what you want to do and prevents you from behaving as spontaneously as your friends. It can be very tempting simply to ignore your diabetes when you feel like this, and to let your blood glucose level run too high.

This behavior can help you fit in with your friends, but it can make you more vulnerable to infections in the short term and do some damage to your blood vessels in the long run.

> **Q** **Can having diabetes stunt your growth?**
>
> **A** Provided your diabetes is well controlled, it should not affect your growth. However, if your blood glucose level is consistently high, you may not reach your full height because your growth hormone will not work effectively if there isn't enough insulin in your bloodstream. This is one reason why you need to keep your blood glucose level within the recommended range as much as possible.

> You might become a bit bored or fed up with testing and injections … however, it's important to find ways to keep going with your diabetes care.

Lots of different insulins, devices, and testing kits are available that can make life easier for you. Your health professional is there to help you work out the most effective system of treatment for your particular needs. You may need to try out different insulin regimens to find one that suits you (see pp.87–90).

Dealing with strong feelings

You might find that you have very strong feelings about having diabetes; for example, anger, resentment, or even hate. You might also feel upset or guilty. These emotions are normal, especially if you have recently found out you have diabetes. But if you think that your feelings are disrupting your studies, work, or family life, you may need to share them with someone else.

Your health professional will probably ask you how you're feeling when you have checkups and will listen and discuss your feelings with you, or you might prefer to talk to someone else. You might find it easier to talk honestly and openly about your diabetes to a school counselor, youth club leader, a friend, or a friend's parent.

Having diabetes can affect the way you see yourself, too. Because insulin builds up the tissues in your body, it can make you put on weight. There are ways to limit this, for example by eating healthily and being physically active, but you might worry about it a lot. You may think that if you don't take your insulin, you won't have to worry about putting on weight—you may even hope that you'll lose weight as you might have done before your diabetes was controlled. However, this is not a healthy way to lose weight, and your blood glucose level would soon become so high that you might be at risk of diabetic ketoacidosis (see p.113).

When you feel well, you may also wonder if you really do have diabetes and, as a result, you might decide not to take your insulin or to take only part of your dose (doing this will remind you what happens to your blood glucose level without enough insulin). Also, from time to time, you will simply forget your injection because you are busy with something else.

However, there is a huge difference between missing the occasional dose and regularly having insufficient insulin. If you keep missing injections, your raised blood glucose level will be high enough to make you feel ill, cause a serious infection, or result in diabetic ketoacidosis, as well as increase your chances of long-term complications.

Managing stress

Getting things into perspective is important – diabetes is for life, but it's not the only thing in your life. Remind yourself that you are doing the best that you can and a short period in which you take less notice of your diabetes won't do you any harm.

> **My experience**
>
> *"I had acute depression…stopped caring about life. The doctor put it down to the enormous psychological effect of having diabetes, which I had coped with far too well as a teenager."* LOUISE
>
> **COMMENT** It is very unusual for a teenager to have such serious depression, but sometimes it is healthier to react emotionally to having diabetes than not to react at all. Louise recovered fully and now believes that she might have felt better had she rebelled a little at the time rather than passively accepting her diabetes.

Stress management can be useful; for example, deep breathing, stretching, a walk in the fresh air, or listening to your favorite music can all help you feel less pressured.

Talking to your family or close friends about all the things you need to do to look after your diabetes can help you feel as though you are sharing the burden, and perhaps help you think of new ways of fitting your diabetes care into your lifestyle. A local support group for young people with diabetes, where you can share your experiences, gripes, and laughs, might also help you feel less isolated.

If you are feeling anxious or depressed about your diabetes, ask your health professional for advice; you might need help to make you feel better about your diabetes and more positive about looking after it. National diabetes organizations, including the Canadian Diabetes Association, also provide important information and updates on managing and living with diabetes (see p.218).

Eating and drinking

Food and drink play an essential part in keeping your blood glucose under control, preventing hypoglycemia, and helping you grow and develop. Of course, eating and drinking are part of your social life, too. The more you can learn about what constitutes healthy eating and how different foods affect your blood glucose level, the better you can adjust your insulin to suit the food you are eating. No foods are banned when you have diabetes and you don't have to eat special foods, but trying to avoid too many unhealthy foods and making healthy choices overall will help you control your diabetes.

You need to eat carbohydrate-containing foods regularly to prevent hypoglycemia. If your eating pattern is irregular or the amount you eat varies a lot, you might need a flexible insulin regimen so that you can easily adjust your insulin doses. You can discuss this with your health professional, who will help you work out the best regimen for you.

You may find that some foods make it difficult to control your blood glucose no matter what you do with your insulin. Trying different insulins and testing equipment, and experimenting with food and insulin doses will allow you to adapt to different situations (see pp.90–95).

Eating a healthy diet is as important for you as it is for your friends who don't have diabetes, but just as they do, you can still have some of your favorite fast food, burger, pizza,

Chinese food, candy, or dessert. Once or twice you may eat a lot of these foods, such as on vacation, but having them every day means you will be eating a lot of extra calories and fat. If you base your eating on a variety of fresh foods such as bread, cereals, fish, and fruit and vegetables, your everyday meals will be low in fat—and this will protect your heart for the future. You can find out more about different meals and how to eat right on pp.30–43.

Blood glucose control

To have good control of your diabetes, your blood glucose test results need to be within your target most of the time, which will mean that your A1C level (see p.66) will be around 7 percent. You'll have your A1C level tested when you visit your diabetes health professional—it's an important test, so this is a good reason to keep your appointments.

You are unlikely to get all your blood glucose tests in the ideal range, partly because this would mean you have lots of bouts of hypoglycemia and partly because taking insulin by injection won't always keep your blood glucose balanced as effectively as natural insulin does. As a result, some of your test results are likely to be outside the desired range.

To keep your blood glucose level as close to the recommended range as possible, you need to look for patterns of high or low readings and work out why they are happening, so that you can make changes to your food, activity, and insulin doses to get your results back on track. You'll need to do this often during your teenage years because hormones such as epinephrine (adrenaline), cortisol, growth hormone, estrogen, and testosterone, which you produce as you grow and develop, can make your insulin less effective. You will find that you need more insulin at some times than at others. Also, if you're female, you may find that your menstrual periods affect your blood glucose level (see p.136).

If you have a consistently high blood glucose level, you'll feel thirsty, tired, and have to urinate a lot. If you try to keep these symptoms at bay by taking enough insulin, you will be doing a lot toward keeping yourself well for the future.

Your diabetes won't make you less likely to get blackheads, acne, or pimply skin, but a high blood glucose level can make you more susceptible to infections, including skin infections. Therefore, if you do get acne or blackheads, see if keeping your blood glucose level well controlled helps prevent them from getting worse.

Tests and injections

Whatever type of insulin you take, you won't always stay on the same dose because life doesn't always stay the same every day. If you didn't have diabetes, your body wouldn't naturally produce the same amount of insulin each day

---

My experience

"In the past, I haven't always been up to doing lots of monitoring and caring for my diabetes, but at least by going to clinics regularly the professionals were getting some idea about my control, by doing A1C readings and checking my feet, kidneys, heart, and eyes." SHELLEY

COMMENT The reality of diabetes is that you don't always feel that you can keep up with its demands. This is why keeping regular appointments with your health professional is essential so that they can encourage and help you at these times.

---

for precisely this reason. As a result, it's essential that you perform regular blood glucose tests so that you can adjust your insulin according to the patterns of your results. By adjusting your doses properly you will be able to eat different foods and amounts and avoid hypoglycemic reactions and an elevated blood glucose level (for more information on adjusting insulin doses, see pp.90–95).

From time to time you may need to try different insulins, devices, and testing kits to find those that really suit you. New injection devices and glucose testing meters are being introduced all the time —if you choose equipment that you like using, you're far more likely to want to look after your diabetes. Talk to your health professional about the choices available to you.

TESTING YOUR BLOOD GLUCOSE Tests don't have to be obvious or time-consuming. Discreet penlike devices and compact meters that give quick results are widely available.

Try different ways of looking after your diabetes to find a routine that suits you better, but avoid changing too often or too much at once. Don't try a new insulin every week, for example, or change your insulin dose, testing routine, and eating pattern all in the same week. Decide on a specific aspect of your diabetes you would like improve or change, and tackle this first before working on another aspect.

If you have type 1 diabetes, there is one experiment you should never try: stopping your insulin completely —because you can't live without it.

Dealing with hypoglycemic episodes

If you're trying to keep your diabetes well controlled, you will have a hypoglycemic episode from time to time. You may feel tempted to keep your blood glucose level higher than the normal range to avoid this, but this isn't a good idea because it will put

you at risk of complications later. Make sure you carry some form of glucose and identification at all times. If you start to get symptoms of hypoglycemia, take action right away (for more information on hypoglycemic episodes and their treatment, see pp.102–109).

Getting on with your life

There is very little you can't do when you have diabetes. There are very few career options that aren't open to you (see pp.118–119), so you can do just about any course of study or type of work. You can also take part in almost any sport. Regular physical activity is especially good for you if you have diabetes, because it helps your insulin work efficiently, which can mean you need smaller doses. You can also drive if you want to, although there are some regulations and precautions to

JOINING IN
Your diabetes won't affect your ability on the sports field or running track—but you'll need to balance your food intake and insulin so that you can perform at maximum capacity.

be aware of before you take to the road (see pp.120–122).

Whether you go on a school or college trip, participate in a competitive sport, work a night shift, or take an exam, your diabetes will always need some attention. When being physically active, for example, you will need to get the balance right between your food and your insulin, so that you can perform at your best (see pp.56–59).

From time to time you will be sick and because illness affects your diabetes, you'll need to know what to do about it. Your blood glucose level might be quite difficult to control because your body is fighting illness, and you might also be unable to eat and drink as normal (see pp.130–133).

Taking exams

Exams can be stressful. Stress often has an effect on your blood glucose control because the hormones you produce when you are stressed, epinephrine (adrenaline) and cortisol, make your insulin less effective (in the same way as when you are ill or during adolescence). Occasionally, you will find that stress has the opposite effect and makes you more vulnerable to hypoglycemia. Your routine can be different while you are taking exams, too, so you may not be able to eat at your usual times.

Therefore, during exam time, you need to keep a close watch on your blood glucose level by doing a few

extra checks each day and changing your insulin doses when you need to. You also need to be prepared with plenty of hypoglycemia treatments, such as glucose pills or a glucose drink, and make sure the proctors know that you may need to eat something during an exam. If you feel hypoglycemic in an exam, act on it right away before it affects your concentration too much.

Drinking alcohol

Alcohol isn't banned when you have diabetes but it can affect you more severely. If you drink a lot and you have a hypoglycemic reaction, you won't be able to recover normally because your body will be so busy processing the alcohol that it will be unable to replace the glucose in your blood. As a result, you could drop way too low. If you're having a drink, eat some food.

If you've had too much to drink, you'll have difficulty checking your blood glucose level before you go to bed. It's best to aim for a blood glucose level that is above your usual bedtime level, so you may need a bigger bedtime snack than usual—hypoglycemia can happen hours after you've stopped drinking.

It's also important to remember that hypoglycemia and being drunk have similar symptoms, so other people may think you are drunk rather than hypoglycemic, especially if they smell alcohol on your breath, they may not realize that you might have a problem. Therefore, be as

---

Practical tips

DRINKING ALCOHOL SAFELY

- Eat a proper carbohydrate-containing meal before you go out drinking.
- If you can't eat before you go out, make sure you have snacks that contain carbohydrate, such as sandwiches or potato chips, while you are drinking.
- Carry glucose – in drink, gel, or tablet form – with you, in case you become hypoglycemic unexpectedly.
- If you're driving, don't drink any alcohol at all.

If you drink a lot and you have a hypoglycemic reaction, you won't be able to recover normally because your body will be so busy processing the alcohol…

responsible as you can about drinking by eating food to accompany the alcohol and by telling your friends about hypoglycemia and how to treat it if you do get into trouble. The designated driver might be your helper, as well. (For more about the effects on diabetes of drinking alcohol, see pp.38–40.)

Smoking

Having diabetes puts you at risk of circulatory problems, and this risk increases if you smoke. It is easy to say "don't smoke," but you may already have started or find it hard to resist when you are offered cigarettes by your friends. It is very important to know the following facts:

• Nicotine is highly addictive, which means that if you start smoking you'll find it difficult to stop.

• You can get help to stop smoking from national and local services and helplines, or you can ask your health professional for support and advice.

• Smoking increases your chances of having a heart attack, stroke, or amputation in the future

because of the combined effects of smoking and diabetes on your blood vessels.

Recreational drugs

Taking recreational drugs is a bad idea, and is especially so when you have diabetes. Drugs can affect your concentration and your ability to look after yourself properly: you might forget to eat, or eat too much, or forget to take your insulin. If you are with people who are taking drugs, they will not be able to help you if you need it. It's true that this could also happen if you don't have diabetes—but when you do have diabetes, the chances of problems occurring with recreational drugs are far greater.

If you decide that you are going to take any drug, you have to know exactly what you are taking, how it will affect your capability to look after your diabetes and what to do to keep yourself safe. Ask yourself the following questions:

• What effect will the drug have and for how long?

• What will happen if I take the drug and then I have a hypoglycemic reaction or I forget to take my insulin?

• Who will notice or be able to help me if I become unconscious?

• Am I likely to become addicted to this drug or its effects?

• What can I do to make sure that I stay safe?

Drugs impair your coordination and awareness. The risks to your

My experience

"I smoked marijuana one day and asked a friend to remind me to check my blood glucose and make sure I was okay. But I got the munchies at 3am and had a very high glucose level later." JOE

COMMENT Joe describes how taking drugs meant that he was unable to care for his diabetes properly, and had to rely on others or suffer the consequences, such as a high blood glucose level after snacking during the early hours of the morning.

health and your diabetes control are very high.

■ **MARIJUANA** Smoking a joint may make you feel more relaxed at the time, but it can also make you feel jittery and uncomfortable. If you use marijuana, it is easy to lose track of time, and to forget to take your insulin or look after your diabetes. It can also make you feel extremely hungry, so you might find yourself eating large amounts of high-fat and carbohydrate-rich food. If you have forgotten your insulin as well, you could end up with a seriously high blood glucose level.

■ **HALLUCINOGENICS** These drugs, which include LSD and magic mushrooms, send you on a "trip." A trip can be very frightening, and you will lose track of time as well as control of your actions and thoughts. This will make it very difficult for you to do anything to look after yourself and your diabetes.

■ **UPPERS** Drugs like ecstasy, speed, and cocaine cause what feels like boundless energy and confidence, so you dance all night. The result is that you use up a lot of energy. They can also make you very dehydrated, which can be aggravated by drinking alcohol. The combination of using energy and being dehydrated can cause severe hypoglycemia. It's important to counteract a low blood glucose level by eating additional food and drinking extra nonalcoholic drinks. But you might not feel at all hungry under the influence of uppers.

Q I've been told that I can't get pregnant because I have diabetes. Does this mean I don't need contraception?

A No—you are just as likely to get pregnant when you have diabetes as anyone else. And don't believe anyone who tells you that you can't get pregnant the first time you have sex either—this is completely untrue. If you want to find out more about contraception and safe sex, your health professional will be able to advise you.

Sex and relationships

It is up to you when or if you tell a new partner about your diabetes, but if you're in a sexual relationship it may be important to do so. Because sex is a form of physical activity, it could cause you to have a hypoglycemic episode, either at the time or some hours later. You may need to tell your partner about this possibility and keep some glucose within reach.

If you are a woman, contraception is particularly important. Unless you are actively planning to become pregnant, either you or your partner needs to use a reliable form of contraception to prevent you from becoming pregnant by accident (see p.127).

In order to have a successful pregnancy when you have diabetes, you need to prepare very carefully . Getting pregnant when your diabetes control is not very good can affect your baby's development (see pp.138–141). For more information on diabetes, sex, and relationships, see pp.126–127.

> It's up to you when or if you tell a new partner about your diabetes, but if you're in a sexual relationship it may be important to do so.

Moving away from home

Leaving home involves a complete change of routine and responsibility. It can be both exciting and a source of anxiety. You will have to make all the decisions about how you manage your diabetes. Although you might be delighted to have your freedom, it is important for you to remember the following points if you are going to be able to live independently.

● You will be responsible for putting food in your kitchen cabinets. Make sure you have enough carbohydrate foods and hypoglycemia treatments for when you need them.

● Keep hypoglycemia treatments in your room as well as in the kitchen, especially if you share a kitchen. Your hypoglycemia supplies need to be available to you, not to your apartment mates!

● You should tell the friends you see regularly about your diabetes and how they can treat a hypoglycemic reaction, maybe with glucagon (see pp.106–109), in case you cannot treat it yourself.

● If you move to a new area, you'll need to find a doctor, although you may be advised to keep your diabetes care in your home town until you move away permanently. Universities usually have on-site health centers, where you can get prescriptions and healthcare if you are ill. If you have started working, you will need someone to contact if you're ill or you can't manage your diabetes for any reason.

● If you become ill, especially with vomiting and diarrhea, it's important to get medical help sooner rather than later, in order to prevent diabetic ketoacidosis (see p.113).

Talking to other people

Most people, including your potential partners, won't know much about what having diabetes means, and some people, including friends and colleagues at work, might have out-of-date or confused ideas about it. When other people don't understand, it can be frustrating to try to talk to them about diabetes, but at least one friend or colleague with whom you spend a significant amount of time should know something about your diabetes and how to help you if you need it.

Your diabetes is just that—yours. In general, it's up to you who you tell and what you say. What won't help, however, is to pretend that you don't have diabetes at all. It can come as quite a shock to other people if you suddenly have a hypoglycemic

> **Your true friends will be genuinely interested in you and your diabetes and will realize that it doesn't change who you are.**

Q My parents insist that I come home for meals and at injection times. I hate having to rush back when I'm out—what can I do?

A If you plan your mealtimes and/or carry food with you and you take your insulin pen, it won't be necessary to be at home for meals or injections. If your parents can be sure that you'll eat and inject your insulin responsibly, they should give you a bit more freedom.

reaction and they don't know what to do. Your family, some friends, and perhaps your colleagues, teachers at school, or professors and academic advisors at college will all need to know about your diabetes so that they can help and support you when necessary.

Talking to your parents

Your parents or caregivers might cross-question you about whether you've done your tests or injections and be concerned about what you're eating and drinking. You might feel that they are nagging, but usually they are just worried and trying to help you. It's a good idea to find a system that you are all happy with—and that doesn't create family tension. You may need to sit and talk calmly for a while before you and your parents come to an agreement.

Talking to your friends

If you prefer not to talk about your diabetes much, choose the person you confide in carefully and work out in advance what you are going to say. If you haven't told your friends, or you have recently been diagnosed, you might worry that they will think differently about you, especially because your treatment involves blood tests and injections. You won't know how they will react until you tell them.

As with anything unfamiliar or surprising, it may take people a little time to get used to what you need to do to look after yourself, but after a while they'll just accept it.

My experience

"I tell people about my diabetes because I know what I'm capable of and if they can't deal with it, then they have the problem, not me!" JANE

COMMENT You aren't responsible for other people's thoughts about your diabetes and as you feel more confident about your ability to deal with the condition, you will learn to ignore unhelpful comments.

If you feel that your friends respond negatively to your having diabetes, it's worth remembering that some people laugh at or make fun of others when they are unsure or even worried about a situation themselves. Your true friends will be genuinely interested in you and your diabetes However, if you are having to put up with a lot of hassling from other people at school or work, it's very important to report it to your teacher or employer.

CONFIDING IN FRIENDS
Some people with diabetes talk about it to just one or two close friends; others feel relaxed telling more. Who and how many people you decide to talk to about diabetes is entirely your decision.

Possible long-term complications

Managing diabetes requires effort and discipline every day. You may feel unable to cope from time to time, and this can develop into depression. Knowing how to deal with such feelings and what kind of help is available is important.

Having diabetes over a period of years causes physical damage to your blood vessels and nerves. Complications resulting from this damage can affect your eyes, kidneys, feet, and heart—and also cause other conditions, such as sexual difficulties.

You can take practical steps to reduce your risk of developing complications, for example by keeping your blood glucose level within the recommended range; maintaining a healthy weight; eating healthily; being physically active; taking your medication regularly; and going for checkups and other appointments.

Being aware of the signs of complications enables you to catch any problems early. And if you do develop complications, it is useful to know what treatment is available and what your future holds.

Depression

Depression is common in people with diabetes, partly because of the constant pressure of managing the condition and partly because of the future or current threat of long-term complications. Feeling depressed can prevent you from looking after yourself. This is why it's important to recognize the symptoms early and prevent things from getting worse. If you are depressed, you may benefit from counseling and/or antidepressant medication.

Understanding depression

Although depression isn't a direct complication of diabetes in the way that, for example, kidney problems (see pp.196–199) are, depression is very common in people with diabetes. About one in five people who have diabetes suffers from depression.

Depression can be problematic if you have diabetes because when you are depressed you often feel tired and unmotivated and this can prevent you from testing your blood glucose regularly, eating food at the right time, or taking your pills or insulin properly. If you are very depressed, there may be times when you believe that there is no point in looking after yourself.

If you think you may be vulnerable to depression, there are various steps you can take to prevent it or lessen

About one in five people who have diabetes suffers from depression.

its effects. There are also treatments available, including counseling, antidepressant medication, or a combination of both.

Causes
When you have diabetes, you may feel depressed because:
- You have just been diagnosed and you are worried or afraid of the effect diabetes will have on your life.
- You are tired of having to deal with your diabetes every day.
- You feel that your diabetes is out of your control, perhaps because your actions don't seem to be having any effect.
- You need to undergo a major change in your treatment, from pills to insulin, for example.
- You have been told that you have signs of the long-term complications of diabetes.
- You are suffering from the advanced complications of diabetes.

TALKING TO SOMEONE
If you are feeling down, you may find it helpful to share your feelings, either with someone you know or a professional counselor, face-to-face or on the telephone. Talking about your feelings can help you come to terms with them.

Alternatively, you may be depressed about something unrelated to your diabetes, such as a bereavement or the breakup of relationship. In these situations, your diabetes can contribute to your depression because it can seem like an additional burden that you don't have the energy to cope with.

Symptoms and diagnosis

There is a difference between temporarily feeling sad and depression. In the first case, your feelings are short-lived and tend not to have a major impact on your everyday life. When you are depressed, however, feelings of despair and sadness can become so dominant that you no longer feel motivated to continue with your usual activities. You may have a combination of emotional and physical symptoms and changes in your thinking, such as:

- Feelings of sadness, pessimism, or hopelessness
- Loss of interest in your usual activities and relationships
- Crying spells
- Sleep disturbances
- Loss of appetite
- Worrying about small things
- Fatigue, apathy, and lack of energy
- Difficulty concentrating
- Lack of motivation

Your health professional can help you consider how much impact any of the above symptoms are having on your life and whether you need help to deal with them.

My experience

"When I was 14 I became very withdrawn and stopped eating. A health professional diagnosed acute depression as a result of the psychological impact of living with diabetes." SOPHIE

COMMENT Being diagnosed with diabetes can have a dramatic effect on your mind as well as your body. You may need to take more time than you think you need, in order to come to terms with the diagnosis of diabetes and its impact on your life.

"When I've been depressed my diabetes has taken a back seat because I've had no energy. I've made some rash decisions about adjusting my insulin, so my glucose has gone very high or low." SHELLEY

COMMENT A fluctuating blood glucose level can make you feel ill and add to your depression. Acknowledging how you feel and seeking help will enable you to get back on track with your diabetes treatment.

Prevention and treatment

Activities that bolster your sense of self-esteem can help prevent depression. For some people, this may mean regular social contact with friends and family, for others it could mean time alone pursuing an enjoyable hobby—find out what works for you. Being physically active (see pp.52–59) has a positive effect on preventing or dealing with depression because it increases the level of mood-enhancing chemicals in your brain. It can also improve your diabetes control by helping your body use insulin more effectively.

If your negative feelings are related to your diabetes, one of the most effective ways to overcome this is to learn as much as you can about diabetes management and put what you've learned into practice. If you feel in control of your diabetes, you can reassure yourself that you are doing your best to prevent long-term complications.

If, on the other hand, your blood glucose level is erratic and you are vulnerable to hypoglycemia or a constantly raised blood glucose level, you are more likely to feel negative about your diabetes. If you can't control your diabetes in a way that allows you to feel confident about what you are doing, ask your health professional for advice.

Admitting that you are feeling down or not coping is important so that you can take action. You may feel as though you are failing or out of control if you admit to feelings of depression, and this can keep you from getting the treatment you need.

When you first start to feel down, talking to your partner or a friend or family member can help you explore what you are going through. It is important to choose someone who allows you to talk and listens impartially, without giving you advice. Talking about depression may be the first time that your feelings become real to you, and another person's advice or opinion may not be useful at this point. Don't be afraid to ask someone just to listen.

If you feel that your depression is getting in the way of your life and particularly if it is stopping you from managing your diabetes, it's a good idea to talk to a health professional. If you find it hard to talk about your feelings, taking a partner, friend, or family member to a consultation may help. Your health professional may recommend counseling or antidepressants or both.

Even if you are feeling very depressed and unmotivated, keeping your diabetes treatment going is still worthwhile. However, you might decide to set realistic goals about how

Practical tips

DEALING WITH NEGATIVE FEELINGS

- Talk to someone—or even out loud to yourself. Simply acknowledging your feelings can be helpful.
- Do some form of regular physical activity—go for a walk, swim, or bike ride, for example.
- Avoid putting pressure on yourself to do all the things you normally do—take time out from your busy schedule.
- Set yourself small achievable goals each day.

much of your diabetes care you feel able to achieve. For example you might take your pills eight or nine times out of ten or test your blood glucose once or twice a day instead of several times.

■ **COUNSELING** Talking to a trained counselor about your depression can help you develop better coping strategies or a more positive way of thinking. Your health professional can refer you for counseling or you may wish to find your own counselor. Counseling may be one-to-one or group-based and it's important that you feel comfortable with the situation as well as with your counselor—you should feel that you can relate to him or her.

Your counselor may use a variety of methods to help you. This will depend on how you are coping emotionally, how anxious you are, and how much your depression is getting in the way of your daily life. For example, you may need help in coping with practical daily activities or you may need to explore the deep emotions you have about diabetes or other aspects of your life. By the time you seek help, you may have been struggling with negative feelings for months or even years, and the issues that arise can take a while to address.

Whatever method your counselor uses, it will help you explore and start to deal with the factors that are causing your depression.

■ **ANTIDEPRESSANTS** Although antidepressants don't take away the underlying reasons for your depression, they can help you cope more effectively. Most antidepressants work by increasing the levels of one or two chemicals in the brain: serotonin and norepinephrine. A variety of antidepressants are available. Most take several weeks to reach their peak effect—this means that you do not start to feel different immediately. You should expect to take antidepressants for a period of at least six months—stopping sooner can mean that your depression is likely to return. The main classes of antidepressants are:

- Tricyclic antidepressants, such as amitriptyline; these work by preventing the resorption and breakdown of serotonin and norepinephrine.
- Selective serotonin reuptake inhibitors (SSRIs), such as fluoxetine; these work by preventing the resorption and breakdown of serotonin.
- Monoamine oxidase inhibitors (MAOIs), such as phenelzine; these work by blocking the activity of an enzyme that can destroy serotonin and norepinephrine.

Outlook

It takes time to recover fully from depression, and the condition can recur. You might still harbor negative feelings for months or even years after a bout of acute depression. Identifying and acting on any symptoms early can help prevent depression from taking over your life.

Myth OR
TRUTH?

MYTH
Depression is always triggered by something.

TRUTH
Tragedy or difficulties can lead to depression, but it can also occur when there is no obvious reason to be sad or negative. Dealing with diabetes every day can cause or contribute to depression, and at times you may need help to cope.

Eye conditions

If you have diabetes, over a period of years the blood vessels at the back of your eyes can become damaged. This is known as retinopathy. At worst, it can lead to loss of sight if untreated. Annual eye examinations are vital to detect and treat problems early, and good diabetes control can prevent the condition from becoming severe enough to affect vision. Cataracts are also more common if you have diabetes and should be monitored and treated to prevent them from affecting your sight.

Retinopathy

The retina is the light-sensitive area at the back of the eye. It receives light, which the optic nerve transmits to the brain, where it is interpreted as a visual image. To function properly, the retina needs a plentiful supply of blood, supplied by a network of small blood vessels.

If you have had diabetes for a long time, your eyes are vulnerable to retinopathy, which is characterized by progressive damage to these blood vessels. Retinopathy can affect one or both eyes.

■ **NONPROLIFERATIVE RETINOPATHY**
During this early stage of retinopathy, also called background retinopathy, blood vessels in the retina bulge and leak blood. On examination of the retina, these bulges, known as microaneurysms, can be seen as small red dots. Other signs of background retinopathy are yellowish spots, known as exudates (consisting of lipoprotein—fat and protein—from leaked blood plasma), and white areas known as "cotton wool spots" in which blood vessels have closed down and stopped supplying the retina with blood. Most people who have had type 1 diabetes for 20 years will have some background retinopathy. Background retinopathy does not necessarily progress further.

■ **PREPROLIFERATIVE RETINOPATHY** The next stage of retinopathy is known as

THE STRUCTURE OF THE EYE
When light enters the eye it is focused by the cornea and the lens on the retina at the back of the eye. Impulses are transmitted by the optic nerve to the brain where a visual image forms. The most sensitive area of the retina is the macula, which contains hundreds of densely packed nerve endings.

Macula

Optic nerve

Retina

Lens

Iris

Cornea

Conjunctiva

preproliferative retinopathy. This is a sign that damage to your eye is progressing. During an eye test, many microaneurysms, exudates, and cotton wool spots can be seen. Also, new blood vessels start to form to replace those that have closed down. These new vessels are fragile and, as a result, are susceptible to leaking and bleeding.

■ **PROLIFERATIVE RETINOPATHY** If preproliferative retinopathy is not treated, more fragile blood vessels form —often on top of your existing blood vessels—and this is described as proliferative retinopathy. The new blood vessels can sometimes bleed into the eye, causing reduced vision.

Causes

Retinopathy can result from a blood glucose level that has been consistently high for a period of years (although retinopathy tends to develop earlier than other long-term complications). High blood pressure can also be a

contributing factor. If you have retinopathy and you become pregnant, the disease may progress more rapidly than it would normally. Also, during pregnancy, previously undiagnosed retinopathy can become apparent

Q **What are my chances of developing retinopathy?**

A Your chance of developing retinopathy increases the longer you have diabetes. If you have had diabetes for 10 years, you have a 50 percent chance of having retinopathy; if you have had diabetes for 20 years, you are almost certain to have background retinopathy. This does not automatically mean that your vision is affected or that it will get worse, it may just mean that there are early signs of damage to your retinal blood vessels. If you have type 2 diabetes, retinopathy may happen on a shorter timescale than this because it may have started to develop before your diabetes was diagnosed. With treatment, you can prevent retinopathy from progressing to a stage at which your eyesight is impaired.

If you have had diabetes for a long time, your eyes are vulnerable to retinopathy.

Practical tips

HAVING AN EYE EXAMINATION

- If you wear glasses, take them along to the test.
- After having eye drops, your pupils will be dilated and unable to contract in bright light—take some sunglasses to wear until the effect of the drops has worn off.
- Don't drive until the effect of the eyedrops has worn off completely and your eyesight is back to normal.

OPHTHALMOSCOPY
The backs of your eyes are examined directly, using a handheld ophthalmoscope, or indirectly, as shown here, using a fixed ophthalmoscope (or slit lamp).

for the first time, so your eyes will be monitored more often.

Symptoms and diagnosis

Retinopathy develops gradually over years and is symptomless until the third stage (proliferative retinopathy) when vision starts to be affected. In severe cases, the complications of retinopathy (see right) may cause partial or complete loss of vision. You should have an eye test to screen for retinopathy when first diagnosed and regularly thereafter. If you already have signs of retinopathy or if you are pregnant, you are asked to have eye tests more frequently. The following tests are used in the diagnosis of retinopathy.

■ **VISUAL ACUITY** This consists of reading rows of letters of diminishing size on a chart known as a Snellen chart. You stand a measured distance away and read the letters aloud, first with one eye covered and then the other. If you wear glasses, you are asked to read the chart while wearing them or to read the letters through a pinhole to see if your detailed vision has changed. If you are unable to read as many lines as at your previous eye test, retinopathy will be suspected and you will have further tests.

■ **RETINAL PHOTOGRAPHY** Your pupils are usually dilated with eyedrops (unless you have a condition known as glaucoma) so that your retina can be viewed clearly. Then a digital or polaroid photograph of your retina is taken and inspected for signs of retinopathy. The advantage of digital photography is that images from consecutive eye tests can be stored electronically, or in your medical records, making them readily available for review and comparison.

■ **OPHTHALMOSCOPY** As with retinal photography, your pupils are dilated with eyedrops. Then your retina is examined using one of two viewing devices: a handheld ophthalmoscope or a fixed ophthalmoscope (also known as a slit lamp). This is done in a very dark room by someone trained in ophthalmoscopy. This examination may be performed in addition to, or instead of, retinal photography to detect the signs of retinopathy.

■ **FLUORESCEIN ANGIOGRAPHY** A dye that is injected into a vein in your arm travels to the blood vessels in your eye. Your retina is then examined under X-ray. Fluorescein angiography is a specialized technique that isn't part of a routine eye test. It may be carried out if you have advanced retinopathy and it is necessary to establish the exact area of the retina that requires laser treatment.

Complications of retinopathy

The following complications of retinopathy can cause severe visual impairment and loss of vision. However, all of them can be avoided if retinopathy is detected and treated from an early stage.

■ **MACULOPATHY** The macula is a central region of the retina that plays a critical role in vision. Retinopathy around the macula—known as maculopathy—may threaten your eyesight. It is more common if you have type 2 diabetes. There are three types of maculopathy.

• Ischemic maculopathy: small blood vessels are damaged and no longer supply blood to the macula.

• Exudative maculopathy: deposits of lipoprotein accumulate around the macula.

• Macular edema: fluid leaks from your blood vessels and gathers around the macula.

■ **VITREOUS HEMORRHAGE** If you have proliferative retinopathy and a large amount of bleeding takes place from the new, fragile blood vessels that have formed in your retina, this is known as a vitreous hemorrhage. You may suddenly lose a large part of your vision, although this is temporary and the blood is gradually resorbed.

■ **RETINAL DETACHMENT** After a vitreous hemorrhage, the blood vessels in your retina form a web that can contract and cause your retina to tear or detach from its base. Retinal detachment may happen a few weeks after a vitreous hemorrhage and can cause permanent damage to your vision.

■ **RUBEOTIC GLAUCOMA** If you have proliferative retinopathy and the new blood vessels in your eye start to grow around your iris, this causes a painful condition known as rubeotic glaucoma. This can cause visual impairment.

Prevention and treatment

The best way to prevent retinopathy from developing or progressing is good long-term blood glucose control, and, if you have high blood blood pressure, managing this correctly (see pp.206–208). It is also important to attend your appointments for eye examinations. If you have retinopathy and a high blood glucose level that suddenly falls because you have started exerting tighter control over your diabetes, your retinopathy may worsen due to changes in blood vessel structure. Improving your blood glucose level over a period of months rather than weeks can prevent this.

Treatment of retinopathy depends on how advanced the condition is. In the early stages of retinopathy (background retinopathy), you don't need any treatment, but your eyes need to be examined for any signs of deterioration regularly.

Blood vessels
Optic disc

Healthy retina

Exudates and fibrous tissue
Optic disc

Blood vessels

A retina affected by proliferative retinopathy

THE RETINA
The ophthalmoscope's view of a healthy retina shows a network of healthy blood vessels extending from the optic nerve. In the retina affected by proliferative retinopathy, blood supply is greatly impeded and the retina is partially covered by fatty exudates and fibrous tissue.

My experience

"Twelve years ago, after 30 years of diabetes, I developed retinopathy and had hemorrhages in both eyes. It was a big shock. I work much harder to control my diabetes now." JOE

COMMENT If you have retinopathy that has been treated satisfactorily or you are in the early stages of retinopathy, maintaining good control of your blood glucose level and blood pressure can prevent problems recurring in the future or progressing to the next stage.

If you have a later stage of retinopathy (preproliferative or proliferative retinopathy), you are given laser treatment. It is not necessary to be admitted to the hospital for this; the treatment can be performed at a specialist outpatient clinic. The procedure consists of directing laser beams at the damaged areas of your retina, in order to destroy the fragile blood vessels that have formed. If you need a lot of laser treatment, this might take place over several visits. Laser treatment carried out during pregnancy does not harm your unborn baby.

Laser treatment is also used to treat maculopathy (with the exception of ischemic maculopathy, which cannot be treated). You can also have laser treatment after a vitreous hemorrhage, but only after the blood has been resorbed by your body—it isn't possible to get a clear view of your retina before this. Laser treatment can prevent deterioration in your vision but cannot restore lost vision.

Sometimes eye surgery may be recommended to treat vitreous hemorrhage and retinal detachment.

> If you receive treatment for retinopathy and your condition stabilizes, the amount of time between your eye examinations can gradually increase.

Although surgery can help restore much of your vision, it does not restore it completely because of the extensive damage that has already occurred to your retina. Surgery might also be used to relieve the pain of rubeotic glaucoma.

If you are treated for retinopathy and your condition stabilizes, the amount of time between your eye examinations can gradually increase until the point at which you only need to attend appointments every six months or yearly. If any problems develop in the future, you are referred back to your ophthalmologist for further investigation and treatment.

Outlook

Retinopathy can be successfully treated. Complete loss of vision can be prevented by good diabetes control, regular and thorough monitoring, and prompt surgery or laser treatment.

Cataracts

If you have diabetes, you are more vulnerable to the development of cataracts, in which the lens of the eye, normally clear, becomes cloudy.

Causes

Cataracts occur as a result of structural changes to protein fibers within the lens. Changes in the protein fibers are a normal part of aging—which is why people who don't have diabetes can also develop them—but they can also be caused by a blood glucose level that has been high for many years.

Symptoms and diagnosis

The cloudiness of the lens prevents sufficient light from entering the eye, resulting in a partial loss of vision. Also, bright lights may appear to have a halo. Because cataracts are progressive, they cause a gradual deterioration in vision (not complete sight loss, as light enters the eye even when cataracts are advanced). Cataracts are diagnosed with an ophthalmoscope (see p.192).

Prevention and treatment

You can reduce your risk of developing cataracts by maintaining good long-term control of your blood glucose. Cataracts can be surgically removed under local anesthetic and a new lens will be inserted.

Outlook

Cataracts develop slowly and may never reach the stage at which they require surgical treatment. If you have surgery, however, your vision will be completely restored.

MATURE CATARACT
Changes to protein fibers in the eye cause the lens to become increasingly opaque. Over time, this causes vision to deteriorate. Cataracts can be treated successfully with surgery.

Living with reduced vision

If your vision is adversely affected by retinopathy or cataracts, making adjustments in your life will enable you to cope. You are entitled to a range of benefits and support to help you do this. To find out more, contact a national organization that works on behalf of people with reduced vision (see p.218).

Impaired vision can affect your ability to manage everyday tasks, and specifically those that are related to your diabetes. If testing your blood glucose level, taking pills, and/or injecting yourself with insulin is difficult, ask your health professional about equipment that can make things easier; for example, a blood glucose meter that has a memory (so that someone else can read your results at a convenient time) or an insulin delivery device with a fixed dose.

Hypoglycemic episodes (see pp.102–109) can be problematic if you have impaired vision because you may not be able to see well enough to treat yourself. You can ask someone close to you for help if you find such tasks difficult or talk to your health professional if you are worried about managing your insulin dosage.

If you drive, you may need to take an eye test, including a field of vision test, to establish whether it is safe for you to continue driving. A field of vision test measures the size of your area of vision on each side (this should be at least 120 degrees).

Myth OR TRUTH?

MYTH
Blurred vision is always a sign of retinopathy.

TRUTH
Blurred vision can be a symptom of a temporarily raised blood glucose level. If your vision becomes blurred, check your blood glucose level and if it is high, take measures to correct it—you may need to adjust your pill or insulin dosage. Your vision should correct itself up to 6 weeks after your blood glucose has improved. In this circumstance, blurred vision is not a sign of retinopathy and provided you continue to keep your blood glucose level in check, should not lead to any long-term problems.

Kidney conditions

Kidney damage, which may occur when you have had diabetes for many years, is known as nephropathy. Symptoms rarely occur until the damage is extensive, so urine and blood tests are used to detect problems early. Good control of blood glucose and blood pressure can prevent it from progressing to a stage where large amounts of protein are lost in the urine, which can indicate kidney damage leading to end-stage renal failure, requiring dialysis or a kidney transplant.

THE KIDNEYS
Each kidney contains about a million mini filtering units, called nephrons, each of which contains a cluster of capillaries (glomerulus), which filter blood, and a long tube called the renal tubule, which resorbs beneficial substances.

Glomerulus

Renal tubule

Nephron

Renal artery

Renal vein

Ureter

Nephropathy

The kidneys filter the blood and get rid of waste products by making urine. They also regulate the amount of fluid and salts in the body, thereby helping control blood pressure. The kidneys' main filtering units are called nephrons. Nephropathy, also known as renal disease, progressively reduces the kidneys' ability to function properly, which causes illness and sometimes leads to kidney failure. The condition develops slowly over a period of years, affecting about 3 in 10 people who have had diabetes for more than 15 years.

■ **MICROALBUMINURIA** In the earliest stage of nephropathy, known as microalbuminuria, tiny amounts of a protein called albumin are found in the urine. This is a sign of early

kidney damage, which can be reversed with treatment.

■ **PROTEINURIA** If the condition worsens, proteinuria, which means an abnormal quantity of protein in the urine, can develop and if protein is consistently present, it indicates that the kidneys have sustained permanent damage. You can have proteinuria temporarily if you have a kidney or bladder infection, and the excess protein disappears when the infection clears up and is not linked to permanent kidney damage.

■ **END-STAGE RENAL FAILURE** Untreated proteinuria can lead to end-stage renal failure—the kidneys can no longer function properly and dialysis or a kidney transplant are required.

Causes

Nephropathy occurs as a result of a high blood glucose level over a period of years, which causes damage to the nephrons. High blood pressure can cause further damage to the kidneys. The first part of the nephron to be affected is a cluster of tiny blood vessels, called the glomerulus. These blood vessels become blocked and leaky, causing protein to escape into the urine and some waste products to remain in the blood. Over time, the filtering tubule in the nephron also becomes damaged, and increasing amounts of protein are excreted in the urine.

If you have had type 1 diabetes for 20 years, you have a 30 percent chance of developing nephropathy. If you haven't developed nephropathy after 30 years, however, you are unlikely to do so. Less is known about type 2 diabetes and the risk of nephropathy, but if you have type 2 diabetes and you also have high blood pressure, or if you are of South Asian descent, your chances of developing nephropathy are significantly increased.

Symptoms and diagnosis

Microalbuminuria does not produce any symptoms, which is why your health professional will carry out urine tests regularly for signs of early kidney damage. A single positive test for microalbuminuria does not necessarily indicate kidney damage: a urine infection can also cause levels of microalbuminuria to rise. For this reason, if a single test is positive, you will have follow-up tests. To confirm the presence of nephropathy, patients are asked to undergo up to two further random urine tests to determine their albumin to creatinine ratio.

If you develop proteinuria, your kidneys are no longer able to filter out waste products or remove excess fluids efficiently. When these build up in your body, they can cause fluid retention, such as swollen ankles or legs, shortness of breath, fatigue, nausea, and itchy skin. Sometimes, however, proteinuria produces no

Myth OR
TRUTH?

MYTH
Once you start to develop nephropathy, it can only get worse.

TRUTH
If nephropathy is treated at the earliest stage, when only very small amounts of protein are present in the urine, your kidneys can recover completely and function normally again. Excellent control of blood glucose levels and blood pressure are essential to avoid further damage.

HEMODIALYSIS AND PERITONEAL DIALYSIS

There are two forms of dialysis: hemodialysis, in which a kidney machine filters the blood, and peritoneal dialysis, also known as continuous ambulatory peritoneal dialysis (CAPD), in which the peritoneal membrane is used as a filter. The type of dialysis you have depends on your health, personal preference, and what is available locally. Your health professional will discuss your options with you.

PROCEDURE	HEMODIALYSIS	PERITONEAL DIALYSIS
How it works	Blood is pumped by a machine through a filter attached to the side of the machine. Inside the filter, waste products and water pass from the blood into dialysis fluid, and the filtered blood returns to the body.	The peritoneal membrane surrounding the abdominal organs is used to filter blood. Dialysis fluid is infused into the peritoneal cavity via tubing attached to a catheter in the abdominal wall. It is drained out a few hours later and replaced with fresh dialysis fluid.
Preparation before starting treatment	Surgery is needed before treatment can start, to connect an artery and vein, usually in your arm, so that the dialysis machine can be connected to your circulatory system.	Surgery is needed before treatment can start, to insert a small tube called a catheter in your abdomen. The catheter can be attached to dialysis equipment.
Where dialysis is carried out	Usually at a dialysis center, but some people are able to treat themselves at home.	At home.
Treatment duration/frequency	3–4 hours, 3 times a week.	1 hour, 4 or more times a day.
Other considerations	Hemodialysis can affect diabetes control and cause hypoglycemia, so you will need to monitor your blood glucose and adjust your treatment regularly. Other drugs and changes to your food intake will be necessary.	You may need to alter the dose of any diabetes medication you take because most dialysis fluid contains glucose, which affects your blood glucose level. You will be prescribed other medications and will need to pay attention to your food intake.

> If nephropathy is diagnosed, you need to bring your blood glucose under tight control.

symptoms at all. You may also have a 24-hour urine test, which involves saving all the urine you pass over a 24-hour period in a bottle, which is sent for laboratory analysis to show how much protein you excrete in a day. You will also have a blood test to measure the creatinine and urea in your blood (waste products that your kidneys should excrete). Your kidneys may also be scanned using ultrasound to look for other causes of proteinuria.

The main symptoms of end-stage renal failure usually include swelling of the face, limbs, and abdomen, a greatly reduced volume of urine, severe lethargy, weight loss, headache, vomiting, and very itchy skin. Urine tests and blood tests are used to detect abnormal levels of waste products in these body fluids.

Prevention and treatment
Keeping your blood glucose and blood pressure under control are important ways in which you can prevent nephropathy from developing or progressing. If nephropathy is

diagnosed, you need to bring your blood glucose under tight control. If your blood pressure is high, this can make the condition worse, so you may be prescribed pills to lower your blood pressure. Stopping smoking, losing weight if you need to, cutting down on salt, and eating less fat if you have high fat (lipid) levels also help lower blood pressure. You may also be prescribed ACE (angiotensin converting enzyme) inhibitor pills or angiotensin-receptor blockers (ARBs) to help reduce the amount of protein you lose through your kidneys and slow the progression of the condition. You will then be monitored with regular blood pressure checks, twice-yearly blood and urine tests to check your kidney function, and twice-yearly A1C tests (see p.66) to check your blood glucose control.

If you develop proteinuria, you may be asked to eat less protein and cut down on foods that are high in potassium (for example, potato chips, yeast extract, and bananas) or salt to prevent waste products from building up in your body. You will need to see a specialist dietitian for advice. Your diabetes medication may also need to be changed because some pills, particularly metformin, should not be taken if you have nephropathy.

If you develop end-stage renal failure, the main treatment options are hemodialysis or peritoneal dialysis, both of which take over the functions of filtering waste products from the blood (see box, opposite). You may be offered a kidney transplant,

but this is less likely to be an option if you have severe heart disease. A kidney transplant also depends on finding a suitable organ donor, and you will need dialysis in the meantime.

If you take pills for your diabetes, you will probably need to change to insulin injections instead. This is because your kidneys are no longer able to excrete diabetes pills, so they will build up in your body and make you more vulnerable to hypoglycemia or other side effects. For the same reason, if you already take insulin, you may need smaller doses than before to control your blood glucose level. You will receive advice from a specialist dietitian about which foods are recommended and which may need to be avoided when you have renal failure. You will also need to limit your fluid intake, possibly to no more than one liter per day.

Outlook

Nephropathy can be successfully treated in the early stages, especially microalbuminuria, and tight control of your blood glucose and blood pressure can reduce your risk of developing nephropathy, slow down, or even halt its progression. If you develop end-stage renal failure, however, the damage is irreversible. You will need dialysis, or a kidney transplant if this is a suitable option for you.

HEMODIALYSIS
If you develop end-stage renal failure, you will need dialysis or a renal transplant. Dialysis involves being connected by tubing to a machine that filters waste products from your blood.

Foot conditions

When you have diabetes, foot conditions can be caused by damage to the nerves in your legs (peripheral neuropathy) or by reduced blood flow to your feet (peripheral ischemia). If you have either or both of these conditions, you are more susceptible to associated complications, such as foot ulcers, Charcot foot, and severe infections, such as gangrene. Knowing the risks, checking your feet daily, and promptly seeking help for any concerns you have can prevent problems from arising.

At least once a year, you need an examination to identify whether your feet are affected by peripheral neuropathy.

Peripheral neuropathy

Damage to the nerves supplying the extremities of your body is known as peripheral neuropathy. The condition, which causes pain or loss of feeling in the toes and feet, can occur in anyone who has had diabetes for several years. If you have type 2 diabetes, you may already have peripheral neuropathy by the time you are diagnosed with diabetes. Peripheral neuropathy may affect a small part of one foot, parts of both feet, or all of both feet. It can also affect your lower legs. Rarely, it can affect your arms and hands.

Causes

Periods of high blood glucose and high blood pressure (see pp.206–208) over months and years cause damage to nerves all over your body. The nerves supplying your feet and lower legs are very long, so if they become damaged and less efficient, these

parts of your body will be affected first. In addition, your feet are particularly vulnerable because they carry your entire body weight and have a great deal of pressure on them.

Symptoms and diagnosis

Symptoms of peripheral neuropathy may include:
- A tingling, burning, or prickling sensation (you might feel pins and needles, for example)
- Short, stabbing, or burning pains, which can be very severe and often occur at night
- Numbness or insensitivity to temperature or pain
- Extreme sensitivity to touch (even a light touch, such as bedclothes lying on your feet at night)

You might have no symptoms at all, or you may experience symptoms and find that they change over time, because nerve damage gradually reduces the feeling in your feet. At

CARING FOR YOUR FEET
When you have diabetes, it is very important to have a daily routine of washing, drying, moisturizing, and checking your feet for any signs of pressure or redness. Keeping your toenails clipped is also important.

least once a year, you need an examination to identify whether your feet are affected by peripheral neuropathy. The health professional examining your feet can tell you whether parts of your feet have reduced feeling. Your feet are examined for:

- Any areas of altered sensation
- Reddened areas that suggest pressure from your shoes
- Very dry skin
- Hard skin (callus) beneath which ulcers (a complication of peripheral neuropathy, see pp.204–205) can form.
- Abnormal warmth
- Wounds or open sores
- Any deformities or change in the shape of your foot due to weakening of your foot muscles

To assess your sensation, your health professional uses various different pieces of equipment, such as cotton wool, a sharp instrument called a neurotip, a nylon filament called a monofilament, or a vibration tuning fork to touch areas of your feet. You are asked whether you are able to feel each touch in order to identify any areas of your feet that have reduced feeling. Your health professional also checks the two pulses in each of your feet, one on the top of your foot, and the other behind your ankle bone. A faint or absent pulse may suggest another condition called peripheral ischemia (see pp.202–204), which can occur in conjunction with neuropathy. You may also have your ankle and knee reflexes tested because peripheral neuropathy can cause muscle weakness and loss of these reflexes.

Prevention and treatment

You can prevent peripheral neuropathy or stop it from getting worse by good blood glucose control. Taking meticulous care of your feet can help identify any problems at an early stage (see pp.128–130).

CARING FOR YOUR FEET

- Check your feet daily for sores or wounds.
- Keep the area between your toes dry.
- Use an unperfumed moisturizer every day.
- Avoid wearing shoes that are too tight.
- Check your shoes for any stones or sharp objects.
- Don't put your feet directly on hot sand, radiators, or a hot-water bottle.
- Avoid using corn plasters or other dressings that contain chemicals.
- If hard skin (callus) starts to build up, have it assessed by a health professional.

If you have peripheral neuropathy, you have a higher risk of damaging your feet through everyday activities. Ask your health professional which parts of your feet have reduced sensation and where problems might develop as a result. Even if you have no soreness or discomfort, it is vital to check your feet daily for pressure areas or constant redness, which could, in time, lead to an ulcer. Talk to your health professional in advance about how to get help, so that you can act quickly if you need to.

If you have painful peripheral neuropathy, you may be prescribed pills to help relieve the pain. You may be given antidepressants or other drugs found to be effective in reducing pain from neuropathy, such as carbamazepine, mexiletine, mild opiod analgesics, gabapentin, or isosorbide dinitrate spray. If your peripheral neuropathy progresses, your pain will gradually reduce as the nerves become more damaged. This makes observation and care of your feet even more important.

Creams that you apply to painful areas can also be helpful. Cream containing capsaicin, an extract of hot chili peppers, is one example, although you should keep it away from open wounds and wash your hands thoroughly after using it. If bedclothes irritate your feet and legs at night, apply a film dressing, or even kitchen plastic wrap, to protect sensitive areas of your feet. You can also obtain a bed cradle to raise sheets away from your feet and legs.

Outlook

Peripheral neuropathy is irreversible, but you can prevent it from worsening by maintaining tight blood glucose control, perhaps by starting insulin injections. Complications associated with peripheral neuropathy are more likely, including foot ulcers (see pp.204–205) and Charcot foot (see p.205). Acute peripheral neuropathy is occasionally resolved by a dramatic improvement in blood glucose control.

Peripheral ischemia

Ischemia is a condition in which the blood supply all over your body is reduced because your arteries are narrowed. Ischemia that affects your legs and feet is known as peripheral ischemia. This condition results in an insufficient supply of oxygen and nutrients to these parts of your body.

Causes of ischemia

Peripheral ischemia is caused by atherosclerosis, in which gradual damage takes place to the inside walls of the arteries. Risk factors for atherosclerosis, and therefore peripheral ischemia, are smoking, a high level of cholesterol in the blood (known as hyperlipidemia), a high-fat diet, and a high blood glucose level over a period of years.

Symptoms and diagnosis

Symptoms usually develop gradually over months or years and include:
- A cramplike pain in your calves following exertion or, less commonly, when you are inactive

• Cold, pale feet
• Wounds or injuries that are slow to heal (a lack of blood flow to your feet deprives wounds of the oxygen and nutrients they need to heal properly)
• Persistent foot ulcers

You may not experience any symptoms at all, but peripheral ischemia can be diagnosed during a foot examination as part of your annual checkup (see p.26). Your health professional assesses the feeling in your feet and checks your foot pulses (faint or absent pulses are a sign of ischemia). If the sensation in your feet is reduced, it suggests that you may have a condition called peripheral neuropathy (see pp.200–202), which often occurs in conjunction with peripheral ischemia. If you are diagnosed with peripheral ischemia, you may be referred for a number of additional investigations, including blood tests, ultrasound scans, or special X-rays, in order to assess how efficiently blood is flowing through your blood vessels.

Prevention and treatment

Healthy eating, regular physical activity, and quitting smoking all help prevent peripheral ischemia. Taking any medication you are prescribed to control blood glucose and blood pressure also reduces risk and helps prevent peripheral ischemia from getting worse.

If peripheral ischemia is mild, regular checkups by your health professional combined with lifestyle changes, in particular, stopping smoking, may be suggested. If the condition is severe and the blood flow to your feet is seriously reduced, you may need surgery. Affected arteries can be widened using a technique called angioplasty, in which a small balloon on the tip of a tube is passed into the artery and inflated. You may need surgery to bypass damaged blood vessels. If the blood supply to your foot is blocked and this cannot be rectified with surgery, or if your foot becomes infected and will not heal, or if gangrene (see p.205) develops, you may need an amputation of part or all of your affected foot.

CHARACTERISTICS OF FOOT CONDITIONS

Peripheral neuropathy and ischemia cause different problems and have different characteristics. However, it is possible to have a combination of the conditions, known as neuroischemia, which further increases your chances of developing foot problems.

PERIPHERAL NEUROPATHY	PERIPHERAL ISCHEMIA
Warm skin	Cool or cold skin
Lack of feeling in foot or feet	Normal or slightly reduced feeling
Pink or normal color	Pale or blue-tinged color
May be painless, but pain can occur and is most severe at night	Painful during exertion or rest at any time of day
Normal or increased pulses in the feet	Faint pulses in the feet, or no pulses at all
Callused skin	No callus
Reduced reflexes	Normal reflexes
Prone to ulcers on any areas of pressure, for example, the soles of the feet	Prone to ulcers on the sides of the feet
Potential to develop Charcot (misshapen) foot	Potential to develop gangrene

Outlook

Peripheral ischemia is irreversible, but it can be stabilized or treated to improve blood flow. You may need some treatments, for example, bypass surgery, more than once. Making lifestyle changes to limit further blood vessel damage is important. You will always be susceptible to associated complications such as foot ulcers, Charcot foot, and gangrene.

Complications of peripheral neuropathy and ischemia

The following complications of peripheral neuropathy and/or peripheral ischemia can cause severe infection, foot deformity, and a loss of blood supply to your feet, which, eventually, can make amputation necessary:

■ **FOOT ULCERS** A complication of peripheral neuropathy, or ischemia, or both, foot ulcers need immediate attention to prevent serious infection.

They are more likely to develop on the soles of your feet or on any areas of increased pressure if you have peripheral neuropathy, and on the sides of your feet if you have peripheral ischemia. Ulcers can develop beneath a layer of callused skin, or be caused by an injury, such as walking on a sharp object, a burn, or a blister resulting from tight or rubbing footwear.

Ulcers do not always hurt, so if you can see any broken or callused skin on one or both of your feet, contact your health professional as soon as possible. In untreated ulcers, layers of skin and underlying foot tissue are gradually destroyed, creating a hole that may sometimes go as deep as your bone. If this happens, you are at risk of developing osteomyelitis (a bone infection). If you have peripheral ischemia, there is a risk that your ulcer may become gangrenous (see p.205).

Ulcers need to heal from their deepest point under the skin outward, so your health professional will remove skin or pus above the ulcer and clean out any dead or infected tissue inside. Your ulcer will then be dressed to protect against infection.

It is vitally important to avoid putting any pressure on your ulcer while it is healing. Walking on an ulcer can make it larger and force an infection deeper into your foot. Your health professional may put a special shoe or cast on your foot to protect it and remove pressure. You might need to wear this for up to 12 weeks to allow the ulcer to heal completely.

Your health professional will take a swab from the wound, which is analyzed in a laboratory to find out whether you have an infection and which type of antibiotics will best treat it. You may be asked to take a long course of antibiotics, possibly for up to eight weeks, to ensure that your infection is controlled (you may need more than one long course of treatment). If your ulcer is severely infected, you may need to stay in the hospital to take all the pressure off your ulcer and have intravenous antibiotics. If an abscess forms, you may need an operation to drain the abscess. An infection that is very deep or will not heal may mean that part of your foot needs to be amputated so that infection is prevented from spreading.

Ulcers take a very long time to heal, but once your ulcer heals, you will need to treat your foot extremely carefully to prevent it from returning; scar tissue at the site of an ulcer can break. Good blood glucose control is important if you have an ulcer or are vulnerable to ulcers, since it reduces the chances of infection (a high blood glucose level makes your body less able to fight infection).

■ **CHARCOT FOOT** This is a complication of peripheral neuropathy, in which the bones of the feet become damaged. Your bone thickness is reduced by neuropathy and a small injury to your foot can cause the bones to quickly fracture or disintegrate. This can dislocate your foot joints. New bone forms at the site of the damage and, as a result, your foot becomes misshapen.

Early signs of Charcot foot are a hot, swollen foot that gets worse over 2–3 months, and might be painful or ache. Treating Charcot foot involves keeping the weight off affected parts of your feet, usually by wearing a cast in the short term and specially made footwear in the longer term. If you have Charcot foot, your foot will change shape over time, so shoes that fit you one day might not fit properly in six months' time. Wear shoes made from flexible material, such as leather, and with adjustable fastenings, such as laces, so that they can adapt to the shape of your foot as it changes. The process of new bone formation will slow and stop after a few months, but permanent deformities will remain.

■ **GANGRENE** This is a complication of peripheral ischemia, in which an area of your foot loses its blood supply altogether. If the blood supply to any part of your foot is cut off, such as to a toe or heel, the skin turns a bluish purple color and then black. Once a toe or foot has developed gangrene, an amputation is necessary to prevent the gangrene from spreading further. If you have had ulcers and pain in your leg for years, an amputation before gangrene develops may improve your quality of life, because it enables you to live without pain.

Cardiovascular conditions

Diabetes is strongly linked to high blood pressure and hyperlipidemia. In addition to being cardiovascular (heart and circulatory) conditions in themselves, they are also major risk factors for other such conditions, for example, coronary artery disease, stroke, and peripheral vascular disease. Identifying your individual risk factors and making appropriate changes to your lifestyle will help prevent cardiovascular conditions from developing.

High blood pressure

When arteries are stiff and narrow, blood is forced through a smaller space at a high pressure—this is high blood pressure (hypertension).

Because high blood pressure is a major cause of other complications of diabetes, such as eye conditions (see pp.190–195), kidney conditions (see pp.196–199), coronary artery disease, stroke, and peripheral vascular disease, prevention and treatment of high blood pressure are essential. Cardiovascular disease is the main cause of death in people with type 2 diabetes. About 10–30 percent of people with type 1 diabetes and 30–60 percent of people with type 2 diabetes have high blood pressure.

Heart

Artery

Vein

THE CARDIOVASCULAR SYSTEM
Blood is pumped by the heart through a dense network of arteries and veins. Arteries carry oxygen-rich blood from the heart to tissues all over the body. Veins carry blood back to the heart.

Causes

Although the link between high blood pressure and diabetes is not yet fully understood, high blood pressure is thought to be partly caused by a high level of insulin circulating in the blood due to insulin resistance in type 2 diabetes or insulin treatment in type 1 diabetes. As a result, blood vessels become scarred, and hard plaques form. In type 1 diabetes, high blood pressure often occurs if your kidney function starts to deteriorate; in type 2 diabetes it is linked with hyperlipidemia and central body obesity. Lack of physical activity, smoking, high alcohol consumption, and stress are also risk factors.

Symptoms and diagnosis

High blood pressure rarely produces symptoms. If you have diabetes and a blood pressure of 130/80 millimeters of mercury (mm Hg) or above when you are tested on several occasions,

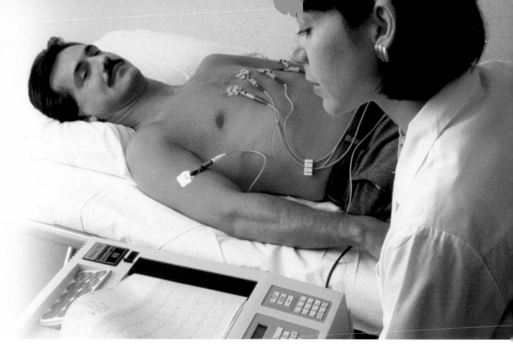

HEART MONITORING
Electrocardiography (EKG) is used to record the electrical activity of the artery and to diagnose abnormal heart rhythms or to investigate the cause of chest pain.

you are diagnosed with high blood pressure. The first figure in a blood pressure reading refers to the pressure when your artery contracts (systolic pressure), the second figure refers to when your heart relaxes between beats (diastolic pressure).

Prevention and treatment

There are very important steps you can take to prevent high blood pressure:
- Achieve and maintain a healthy weight.
- Limit alcohol consumption.
- Limit sodium intake.
- Quit smoking.

Maintaining good blood glucose control and keeping your alcohol consumption within normal limits also helps. If you have been diagnosed with high blood pressure, reducing your salt intake can be helpful.

If your blood pressure is high on several occasions, you will receive treatment and be reviewed every three to six months. The following pills are used to treat high blood pressure (you may need to take up to three different types of pill).
- Angiotensin converting enzyme inhibitors (ACE inhibitors) work by dilating your arteries.
- Angiotension-receptor blockers (ARBs) lower blood pressure and reduce your risk of cardiovascular events.
- Cardio-selective betablockers work by blocking the action of epinephrine (adrenaline), a hormone that increases your heart rate and raises blood pressure.
- Diuretics (used in low doses) work by decreasing the volume of fluid in your body and dilating your arteries, thereby reducing your blood pressure.

Outlook

If your blood pressure is maintained at 130/80 mm Hg or below, either by changes in your lifestyle or by taking

Practical tips

QUITTING SMOKING SUCCESSFULLY

- Try nicotine skin patches or nicotine chewing gum.
- Go to a quit-smoking clinic.
- Change your routine and associations. For example, if you always smoke after a meal, go for a walk after meals instead.
- Socialize in places where you can't smoke, such as the movies instead of a bar, or the non-smoking section of a restaurant.
- If you feel you can't stop completely, start by cutting down to one or two cigarettes a day.

pills, this greatly reduces your risk of developing coronary artery disease, stroke, peripheral vascular disease, and eye and kidney conditions.

Hyperlipidemia

An abnormally high level of fats (lipids) in the blood, referred to as hyperlipidemia, is a major cause of coronary artery disease, stroke, and peripheral artery disease. It is more common in people with type 2 diabetes. If you have type 1 diabetes, you are likely to have normal levels of fats in the blood unless there is another reason for the levels of fats to be raised.

Causes

The link between diabetes and hyperlipidemia isn't fully understood, but the abnormally high level of insulin caused by insulin resistance in type 2 diabetes is thought to be partly responsible. If you have type 2 diabetes, you are more likely to develop the condition if you are obese and have high blood pressure. Other general risk factors in either type 1 or type 2 diabetes include a high-fat diet, inactivity, smoking, obesity, an underactive thyroid gland, and a high blood glucose level over many years. A high alcohol intake and a family history of hyperlipidemia are also contributing factors.

Symptoms and diagnosis

Hyperlipidemia rarely produces symptoms. At your annual checkup (see p.26) you will have a blood test to measure cholesterol. If the result is high, you are given healthy eating advice. You may be offered more blood tests to find out the levels of triglycerides and low-density lipoprotein (LDL), and your ratio of total cholesterol to high-density lipoprotein (HDL) (see chart, left).

Prevention and treatment

There is much you can do to prevent hyperlipidemia: eating healthily, especially avoiding saturated fats (see p.36), becoming more physically active, and losing weight are very important. Good diabetes control and reducing a high alcohol intake can also help. Treatment consists of pills. Which type you need depends on your blood fat level:

- Statins work by preventing cholesterol production.
- Fibrates work by reducing the production of triglycerides.

Your blood lipid levels may be tested every three to six months to assess whether treatment is working.

HEALTHY LEVELS OF FATS IN THE BLOOD

High levels of some fats (lipids) in the blood—and low levels of others—increase your risk of coronary artery disease. If you have a blood test to check your lipid levels, these are the results that you need to aim for to keep your heart and blood vessels healthy.

TYPE OF FAT	HEALTHY LEVEL
Triglycerides	Below 1.5 millimoles per liter
LDL cholesterol	Below 2.5 millimoles per liter
Total cholesterol to HDL ratio	Below 4

Outlook

If your blood lipid levels remain healthy due to changes in your lifestyle or to taking pills, your risk of developing coronary artery disease, stroke, and peripheral vascular disease is significantly reduced.

Coronary artery disease (CAD)

The two main arteries that encircle the heart and supply it with blood are known as the coronary arteries. If you have diabetes, you have an increased risk of CAD, in which fatty deposits known as atheromas build up in your coronary arteries and restrict blood flow to your heart.

Causes

A high level of insulin may be responsible for damage to the arteries (see High blood pressure, pp.206–208). Other risk factors are high blood pressure, hyperlipidemia, a high-fat diet, inactivity, smoking, obesity, a family history of CAD, and a blood glucose level that has been high for a period of years.

Symptoms and diagnosis

When the heart receives insufficient oxygen because blood flow through the coronary arteries is restricted, you may experience angina, a heart attack, or heart failure.

■ **ANGINA** A temporary sensation of pain or pressure in the chest is the main symptom of angina. You may also experience pain in your left

Q What is my risk of developing a circulatory condition?

A If you have diabetes and your blood glucose level is regularly above 7 millimoles per liter; your A1C test result is above 7 percent; you smoke; you have high blood pressure (above 130/80 mm Hg); a BMI above 30 (see p.46); or you are of African, Latin American, Aboriginal, or Asian descent, you have a significant risk of developing a circulatory condition. Also, if you are a woman with diabetes, you lose extra protection against circulatory problems after menopause. If one or more of the above apply to you, you can still do a great deal to reduce your risk by making changes to your lifestyle, for example, by losing weight, being more physically active, or stopping smoking.

shoulder or down the inside of your left arm. This can happen when you are stressed or you exert yourself, for example, lifting a heavy object or walking faster than usual.

■ **HEART ATTACK** The main signs of a heart attack are severe chest pain, breathlessness, a pounding or irregular heartbeat, sweating, lightheadedness, nausea, and sometimes loss of consciousness. Symptoms may also be mild or absent altogether.

■ **HEART FAILURE** The heart gradually loses its ability to pump blood around the body. Signs of heart failure include swelling in your abdomen, legs, and feet, fluid in your lungs, shortness of breath, and fatigue. The condition usually worsens slowly over time.

CAD may be diagnosed by an electrocardiogram (EKG) in which the heart's electrical impulses are recorded with electrodes placed on

A temporary sensation of pain or pressure in the chest is the main symptom of angina. You may also experience pain in your left shoulder or down the inside of your left arm.

CORONARY ARTERIES
A network of arteries and veins supply blood to the heart so that it can be pumped around the body. Narrowing of the coronary arteries that supply the heart muscle can cause coronary artery disease.

The symptoms of a stroke depend on which part of the brain has been damaged. Your movement, speech, memory, vision, hearing, or balance may be affected.

the skin. Imaging techniques using ultrasound waves and X-rays may be used to view the heart and assess the health of the coronary arteries.

Prevention and treatment

Lifestyle changes are the most important ways of preventing CAD: including eating a healthy diet, being physically active, stopping smoking, losing weight if necessary, reducing alcohol intake, and managing stress. Monitoring your blood pressure and blood lipid levels regularly and getting treatment if necessary will help. You can also help prevent CAD by maintaining good long-term control of your diabetes.

The treatment for CAD consists of drugs or surgery. Some of the available drug treatments have potential uses in controlling blood pressure as well as reducing the risks for cardiovascular disease and nephropathy.

The main surgical treatments for CAD are coronary artery bypass surgery and coronary angioplasty. Bypass surgery involves grafting a blood vessel from another part of your body and rerouting blood away from the damaged part of the artery. Coronary angioplasty involves feeding a fine tube into the blocked part of the artery and inflating a "balloon" at the end of the tube. This widens the artery so that, when the balloon is deflated and removed, blood can flow unimpeded. A metal device known as a stent may also be implanted in an artery to keep it open.

If you have a heart attack and you are admitted to the hospital, you will be treated with an insulin infusion followed by insulin injections at home for several months afterward. This is to reduce your chances of having a further heart attack. You may or may not need to remain on insulin in the longer term, depending on your blood glucose control and other risk factors.

Outlook

There are very good prevention and treatment options for CAD, including pills to reduce the risk of heart attacks. However, a healthy lifestyle remains an important part of keeping your circulation at its most efficient.

Stroke

When the blood flow to your brain is interrupted as a result of a blood clot or a burst blood vessel, your brain is deprived of oxygen and this causes some brain cells to die or be damaged.

Causes

The main risk factor for stroke is high blood pressure, which is a common complication in people with diabetes. Atherosclerosis (associated with high cholesterol in the blood), in which fatty deposits cause narrowing of the arteries, is another risk factor.

Symptoms and diagnosis

Stroke symptoms depend on which part of your brain has been damaged. You might find you have a combination of your movement being affected, as well as your, speech, memory, vision, hearing, or balance. A stroke is likely to be diagnosed by your symptoms, and you may possibly also need a brain scan.

Prevention and treatment

If you have high blood pressure (see pp.206–208), keeping this well controlled by taking medication regularly and following guidelines for a healthy lifestyle can help prevent stroke. Cutting down on saturated fat in food also helps keep your circulation healthy. The treatment for stroke consists of assessment and rehabilitation of the functions affected; this may include physical therapy and speech therapy.

Outlook

The outlook after a stroke depends on the functions that are affected, and how badly. Recovery may be possible with the help of a specialist.

Peripheral vascular disease (PVD)

When fatty deposits build up in the arteries in the arms or legs, blood flow is restricted to the arm and leg muscles. This is known as peripheral vascular disease (PVD).

Causes

A high level of insulin circulating in the blood may be responsible for damage to the arteries (see High blood pressure). Other risk factors are high blood pressure, hyperlipidemia,

a high-fat diet, inactivity, smoking, obesity, and a blood glucose level that has been consistently high for a period of years.

Symptoms and diagnosis

The first sign of a narrowed arm or leg artery is pain and fatigue in the arm or calf muscles during physical activity caused by restricted blood flow (the greater the exertion, the greater the pain). PVD is diagnosed by your symptoms and history plus X-rays or ultrasound scans.

Prevention and treatment

The best way to prevent PVD is to combine healthy eating and physical activity with good long-term control of your diabetes. It can help to lose weight if you need to, quit smoking, and reduce your alcohol intake. It's important to have your blood pressure and blood lipid levels monitored and to take any treatment regularly. Treatment of PVD consists of medication that will help reduce the constriction of your arteries and will also prevent your blood clotting too easily. You may also be offered angioplasty or bypass surgery to improve or replace the damaged artery (see p.210).

Outlook

The treatment for PVD, either by medication or by surgery, can be very successful. However, reducing risk factors for further damage, especially by stopping smoking, will enhance their long-term success.

Practical tips

PREVENTING CARDIOVASCULAR CONDITIONS

- Eat a healthy diet, including at least 5 portions of fruit and vegetables daily. Limit saturated fat.
- Do some physical activity, such as brisk walking for half an hour, five times a week.
- Quit smoking.
- Keep your body mass index in the recommended range (see p.46).
- Keep your diabetes well controlled.
- Limit your alcohol consumption if you have been advised to do so.
- Make sure you take any medication you are prescribed to reduce your blood pressure or blood lipid levels.

Other conditions

If you have had diabetes for a long time, you are susceptible to a number of conditions. Lumpy skin at insulin injection sites (lipohypertrophy) can develop if you repeatedly inject in the same site. Erectile dysfunction, also known as impotence, can occur as a result of nerve damage or blood flow problems, while damage to the nerves that control automatic bodily functions, such as your digestion and your body temperature, is known as autonomic neuropathy.

Lipohypertrophy

Lumpy skin at insulin injection sites is known as lipohypertrophy. The lumps are swollen and raised, but not red or painful.

Causes

Repeated injections in the same injection site can cause fat deposits to accumulate under the skin. Insulin can also cause overgrowth of tissues where the skin is damaged. You are more likely to get lipohypertrophy if you use the same sites to inject your insulin for years, but it can develop after using the same site for only a few months.

Symptoms and diagnosis

Lumps usually develop slowly, so you may not notice that anything is wrong. Run your hand across your injection sites to assess whether the skin feels different there. If you can't feel any lumps but your blood glucose level fluctuates from day to day for no

apparent reason, contact your health professional. Unpredictable swings in your blood glucose level indicate that you might be injecting into sites where cell growth is abnormal, which affects the absorption of your insulin. Your health professional will be able to tell you if you have lipohypertrophy by examining your injection sites.

Prevention and treatment

To avoid lipohypertrophy, don't inject into the same area each time (to find out where you can inject see p.97). If you already have lipohypertrophy, don't inject into any lumpy areas, even if injections there seem to feel less uncomfortable. If insulin absorption has been a problem, you may have increased your dose to combat this without knowing that lipohypertrophy was the problem. In this case, you may need to reduce your insulin dose by up to half when you use a new injection site to avoid hypoglycemia.

Myth OR TRUTH?

MYTH
Skin problems at injection sites are inevitable.

TRUTH
You can take steps to avoid skin problems. To prevent bruising, use a short needle to inject. To avoid lipohypertrophy (see right), change injection sites regularly. If you have an allergic reaction to an insulin, however, consult your health professional about changing brands.

Outlook

Over time, the lumps should reduce
in size as fat cells are resorbed into
your body. Large or long-standing
lumps, however, may never disappear
entirely, in which case you should
never use these injection sites again.

Erectile dysfunction

Erectile dysfunction (ED), which is
also known as impotence, is an
inability to achieve or sustain an
erection so that sexual intercourse can
take place. The condition affects about
one in three men who have diabetes
and becomes more common with age.

Causes

Erectile dysfunction occurs as a result
of a high blood glucose level over
many years, which can damage your
circulation and nerves, and lead to
autonomic neuropathy (see p.215).
As a result, the blood supply to the
penis may be affected or nerve damage
can affect the processes leading to
sexual arousal. Erectile dysfunction
may also be a side effect of drugs,
including those used to lower blood
pressure, for example beta blockers.
There are other causes of ED that
may or may not be related to your
diabetes. These include depression,
stress, anxiety, and relationship
difficulties. Your risk of ED is also
increased by heavy smoking and
drinking. Rarely, ED is caused by low
levels of testosterone or the hormone
thyroxine. Discussing your symptoms
and lifestyle with your health
professional will help identify which
physical and/or psychological factors
are involved in your ED.

Symptoms and diagnosis

Your ED is less likely to be diabetes-
related if you have erections during
the night or in the mornings, if your
ED has developed suddenly, or if you

Erectile
dysfunction
affects about one
in three men who
have diabetes.

only suffer from ED in specific situations, such as when you feel stressed or when you are with a new partner. It is more likely to be linked to your diabetes if you are unable to achieve an erection at all and the problem has developed gradually. You may need tests to help identify the cause of ED, including a blood pressure check, physical examination, and a blood test to check testosterone and thyroxine levels. You may be tested for autonomic neuropathy (see right) or for peripheral neuropathy (see pp.200–202) because, if other parts of your body are affected by nerve or circulation damage, diabetes may be a factor in your ED.

Prevention and treatment

The most important step you can take to prevent ED is to control your blood glucose. Initial treatment involves dealing with any underlying cause of your ED, for example if drug treatment is a likely cause, your health professional may suggest changing your medication. Low testosterone or thyroxine levels can also be treated with medication. Tight control of your blood glucose is very important and you may need to increase the dose of your pills or insulin, or take a new medication to achieve this. You should also stop smoking and reduce your alcohol intake if you drink more than the safe amount (see p.38). If these measures do not restore your full sexual function, you may be offered further drug or physical treatments as well as counseling.

ED is more likely to be connected to your diabetes if you are unable to achieve a erection at all and the problem has developed gradually.

■ **DRUG TREATMENTS** The following drugs work by relaxing the muscles around the penis and improving blood flow to produce an erection.
• Alprostadil (Caverject) is inserted into the urethra in pellet form, or injected directly into the penis. Alprostadil can have side effects; your erection may not subside as normal after sexual activity and, if you use the injection form, bruising may occur around the injection site.
• Sildenafil (Viagra) or vardenafil (Levitra) are taken orally about one hour before sexual activity. Viagra can be effective for up to 6–8 hours; Levitra for up to 48 hours. They should not be taken with drugs containing nitrates, such as isosorbide mononitrate or glyceryl trinitrate, which you might be taking if you suffer from angina or high blood pressure, because the two together can cause very low blood pressure.
• Tadalafil (Cialis) is taken orally 30 minutes to 12 hours before sexual activity, and works for up to 36 hours. It should not be taken with nitrates.
• Apomorphine hydrochloride (Uprima) is taken orally about 20 minutes before sexual activity. It is safe to take this drug with nitrates.
■ **PHYSICAL TREATMENTS** There are several physical aids that can help you achieve and maintain an erection. The vacuum device consists of a plastic tube and rubber band that is placed over the penis. You use a pump to create a vacuum inside the tube, causing the penis to fill with blood and become erect. You then

slip the rubber band onto the base of your penis to maintain your erection, and remove the tube and pump.

If blood vessels to your penis have become narrowed, surgery can restore normal blood flow. There is also a variety of penile implants available, from rods that keep the penis erect all the time (you fold your penis against your thigh or abdomen) to an inflatable device that is activated with a pump to hold the penis erect.

Outlook

Most treatments are effective and allow you to continue to enjoy lovemaking. However, they can make sex less spontaneous. Involving your partner in decisions about treating ED and incorporating that treatment into your lovemaking, can make your sex life more enjoyable. You may choose not to have treatment. ED does not adversely affect any other aspect of your diabetes or your overall health.

Autonomic neuropathy

The nerves controlling parts of your body that you don't move voluntarily are the autonomic nerves. They help the body function by regulating your temperature, your heart rate, and your digestive system, for example. When these nerves are damaged, this is known as autonomic neuropathy.

Causes

Autonomic neuropathy is the result of consistently high blood glucose over many years. Damage to the nerves makes them less effective at transmitting impulses, which can affect your body's normal functions.

Symptoms and diagnosis

Autonomic neuropathy can produce a range of symptoms, including:
- Too much or too little sweating, very dry skin
- Nausea, vomiting, diarrhea or constipation.
- Dizziness (postural hypotension) when you stand up or get out of bed
- Difficulty exercising because your heart rate does not increase/decrease
- An inability to empty your bladder completely
- Erectile dysfunction
- Reduced awareness of hypoglycemia

If you have more than one of the above symptoms, see your health professional to have your heart rate and blood pressure checked, as these are also under the control of your autonomic nervous system.

Prevention and treatment

Good blood glucose control helps prevent autonomic neuropathy. Specific symptoms of the condition are treated as they occur. You may be prescribed medication to relieve nausea, vomiting, and diarrhea, for example.

Outlook

Autonomic neuropathy is likely to be permanent, because the nerve damage cannot be repaired; therefore, treatment is aimed at relieving your symptoms as they arise.

Practical tips

AVOIDING POSTURAL HYPOTENSION

- When you get up in the morning, sit on the edge of the bed for 5 minutes before standing up.
- Try keeping your head and shoulders raised while you sleep, perhaps on extra pillows or by adjusting your bed slightly, if you have an adjustable mattress.
- Ask your health professional whether wearing support stockings at night would help relieve your symptoms.

Glossary

A1C (GLYCOSYLATED HEMOGLOBIN) test that measures the level of glucose in the blood over the previous 6–8 weeks.

AUTONOMIC NEUROPATHY damage to the nerves (autonomic nerves) that affect various involuntary body functions such as digestion and body temperature.

BACKGROUND RETINOPATHY the first stage of retinopathy, in which blood vessels in the retina, at the back of the eye, bulge and leak blood; at this stage, some blood vessels have also closed down and have stopped supplying blood to the retina.

BETA CELLS cells in the pancreas that produce insulin.

BLOOD GLUCOSE LEVEL the concentration of glucose (sugar) in the blood, measured as the number of millimoles (mmol) of glucose per liter of blood.

BMI (BODY MASS INDEX) height to weight ratio; the BMI is calculated by dividing your body weight (in kilograms) by your height (in meters) squared.

ERECTILE DYSFUNCTION inability to achieve or sustain an erection for sexual intercourse.

EXTENDED LONG-ACTING INSULIN ANALOGUE a type of insulin that is injected once a day and that provides a background supply of insulin with no peak of action.

FAST-ACTING INSULIN a type of insulin injected 20–40 minutes before mealtimes that peaks within 2–3 hours after injection.

GESTATIONAL DIABETES diabetes developed during pregnancy that disappears after the baby is born.

GLUCAGON a hormone produced by the pancreas that raises the level of glucose in the blood by converting glycogen stored in the liver back into glucose.

GLUCOSE a simple sugar that is the body's primary energy source; most of the body's glucose supply comes from the digestion of carbohydrates and from glycogen stored in the liver being converted back into glucose.

GLYCOGEN the form in which glucose is stored in the liver.

GLYCOSYLATED HEMOGLOBIN see A1C.

HYPERGLYCEMIA a high blood glucose level—above 7 millimoles of glucose per liter of blood.

HYPERLIPIDEMIA high levels of fat in the blood.

HYPOGLYCEMIA a low blood glucose level—below 4 millimoles per liter.

INFUSION fluid or insulin delivered continuously into a vein, usually carried out in the hospital.

INJECTION SITE area of the body where insulin is injected.

INSULIN a pancreatic hormone produced to lower blood glucose by allowing glucose to enter body cells.

INSULIN DEVICE any device that is used to deliver insulin by injection.

INTERMEDIATE-ACTING INSULIN insulin that is injected once or twice daily, which has a peak of action between 4–8 hours after injection, providing a background supply of insulin.

ISCHEMIA reduced blood supply to part of the body, due to narrowing of arteries.

KETOACIDOSIS a serious condition, caused by a very high blood glucose level, in which ketones are produced and the acid balance of the blood is affected.

KETONES acid by-products, produced from the breakdown of fat. Can be highly toxic if there is a severe lack of insulin.

LIPOHYPERTROPHY fatty lumps under the skin caused by repeatedly injecting into a small area of the body.

LIPOPROTEINS substances that consist of a protein combined with fat.

LONG-ACTING INSULIN insulin that is injected once a day and has a peak of action between 6–10 hours after injection, providing a background supply of insulin.

MICROALBUMINURIA very small amounts of protein in the urine; an early sign of nephropathy.

MILLIMOLES PER LITER measure of blood glucose level.

MODY (MATURITY-ONSET DIABETES OF THE YOUNG) diabetes with a specific genetic pattern, similar to type 2 diabetes in its treatment.

NEPHRON the basic filtering unit of the kidney, consisting of a cluster of blood capillaries (glomerulus) and a long, thin tube (renal tubule); each kidney contains about one million nephrons.

NEPHROPATHY reduction in the kidneys' ability to function.

NEUROPATHY damage to the nerve supply in the body.

PANCREAS abdominal organ producing insulin, glucagon, and other digestive hormones.

PERIPHERAL ISCHEMIA reduced blood supply to legs and feet, due to narrowing of arteries.

PERIPHERAL NEUROPATHY damage to the nerves supplying the extremities of the body.

PREPROLIFERATIVE RETINOPATHY the second stage of retinopathy (see Background Retinopathy), in which new blood vessels start to form in the retina to replace those that have closed down; the new blood vessels are fragile and prone to bleeding.

PROLIFERATIVE RETINOPATHY the final stage of retinopathy, in which many new blood vessels form in the retina, often on top of existing blood vessels; the new blood vessels may bleed into the back of the eye, reducing vision.

PROTEINURIA large amounts of protein in the urine, a sign of permanent nephropathy.

RAPID-ACTING INSULIN ANALOGUE a type of insulin injected at mealtimes that peaks within 1–2 hours after injection.

RETINAL DETACHMENT separation of the retina from its underlying layers; retinal detachment is a potential complication of retinopathy.

RETINOPATHY any disorder that affects the retina, usually due to damage to retinal blood vessels.

RUBEOTIC GLAUCOMA a potential complication of proliferative retinopathy in which the new blood vessels in the eye grow around the iris, which can cause visual impairment.

TYPE 1 DIABETES diabetes in which the beta cells in the pancreas have been destroyed and, as a result, the body can no longer produce insulin.

TYPE 2 DIABETES diabetes in which the body cells are resistant to the action of insulin and insulin production gradually declines.

VITREOUS HEMORRHAGE bleeding into the rear of the eye, a temporary condition that is a potential complication of retinopathy.

Useful addresses

The following organizations provide useful information; some also offer support or can help you to make contact with other people who have diabetes. You can also obtain details about further sources of information from your health professional.

Canadian Diabetes Association
1400–522 University Avenue
Toronto, Ontario M5G 2R5
Phone: 1-800-BANTING (226-8464)
Web site: www.diabetes.ca

Canadian Health Network
Web site: www.canadian-health-network.ca

Canadian Institutes of Health Research
160 Elgin Street, 9th Floor
Ottawa, ON, K1A 0W9
Tel: 1-888-603-4178
Web site: www.cihr-irsc.gc.ca

Canadian MedicAlert® Foundation
2005 Sheppard Avenue East, Suite 800
Toronto, Ontario M2J 5B4
Tel: 416-696-0267
Web site: www.medicalert.ca

Diabète Québec
8550 boul. Pie-IX, bureau 300
Montréal, Québec H1Z 4G2
(514) 259-3422
Tel: 1-800- 361-3504
Web site: www.diabete.qc.ca

Dietitians of Canada
480 University Avenue,
Suite #604
Toronto, Ontario M5G 1V2
Tel: (416) 596-0857
Web site: www.dietitians.ca

Health Canada
A.L. 0900C2
Ottawa, Canada
K1A 0K9
Tel: (613) 957-2991
Toll free: 1-866-225-0709
Fax: (613) 941-5366
Web site: www.hc-sc.gc.ca

Juvenile Diabetes Research Foundation International
7100 Woodbine Avenue
Suite 311
Markham, Ontario
L3R 5J2
Tel: (905) 944-8700
Toll free: 1-877 CURE 533
Fax: (905) 944-0800
e-mail: general@jdrf.ca
Web site: www.jdrf.ca

National Aboriginal Diabetes Association Inc.
174 Hargrave Street
Winnipeg, Manitoba R3C 3N2
Tel: 1-877-232-NADA (6232)
Web site: www.nada.ca

National Institute of Diabetes and Digestive and Kidney Diseases
National Institute of Health
Building 31, Room 9A04 Center Drive, MSC 2560, Bethesda, MD 20892
Tel: (800) 860-8747
Tel: (301) 654-3327
Web site: www.niddk.nih.gov

National Kidney and Urologic Diseases Information Clearinghouse
3 Information Way, Bethesda, MD 20892
Tel: (800) 891-5390
Tel: (301) 654-4415
Web site:
http://kidney.niddk.nih.gov

Index

Acknowledgments

Authors' acknowledgments We would like to thank the following people for their support and contributions: Stuart Bootle; Jane, Jake, and Charlie Buckingham; Shelley Foster; Iain, Vicky, Daniel, and Emma Levitt; Steven Sexton; Joe Solowiejczyk; Nick Steiner; Janet Sumner; Sophie Thomas; Graham Toms; George Walker; Jan Williamson; and the staff of The Hollies medical center. We would also like to thank the many others who have contributed along the way, providing information and support at crucial times while we were writing. In addition, the editorial and design teams of Dorling Kindersley and Cooling Brown have been invaluable in helping us understand the world of publishing. We have also received strong support and endless encouragement from our friends, families, and close colleagues. We hope all of you will celebrate and enjoy the final product.

Photographer Trish Gant
Models Charlie Buckingham, Jake Buckingham, Jane Buckingham, Angela Cameron, Sagaren Pillay, Nicholas Steiner, George Walker, Jeremy Wallis, Jan Williamson.
Index Hilary Bird

Picture credits

Alamy: Mark Harmel 6bl; Epictura 136tl; Image100 148tl; Jack Sparticus 157br; Image Source 163tr; Mark Harmel 177br. **Corbis**: John Henley 2; John Henley 19tr; Roy Botterell 30tl; Roy Botterell 31tr; Ronnie Kaufman 47br; Thom Lang 76tl; Jose Luis Pelaez, Inc. 77tr; © LWA—Dann Tardif 103tr; Steve Prezant 111tr; Ford Smith 126bl; Ken Redding 129tr; Mark M Lawrence 137tr; Charles Gupton 165br; 171tr; Kevin Fleming 178b; © LWA—Dann Tardif 184; 206tl. **Dorling Kindersley:** David Murray and Jules Selmes 42bcl; David Murray and Jules Selmes 42br; Simon Brown 154tl; Simon Brown 155tr. **Getty**: Taxi/Stephen Derr 7bc; Image Bank/Romilly Lockyer 8; Taxi/Gary Buss 10tl; Photographer's Choice/Nancy Brown 16bl; Taxi/Gary Buss 23tr; Photodisc Red 26bl; Taxi/Dan Kenyon 28; Photographer's Choice/Robin Macdougall 33br; Image Bank/Garry Gay 36bla; Image Bank/Rita Maas 36bl; Taxi/Antonio Mo 43cra; Stone/Steven Peters 45tr; Image Bank/Sean Justice 52tl; Taxi/Stephen Derr 53tr; Stone/David Madison 55br; Image Bank/Yellow Dog Productions 59b; Taxi/Justin Pumfrey 60; Taxi/Arthur Tilly 66bl; Thinkstock 74b; Image Bank/Marc Romanelli 81br; Image Bank/Daly & Newton 114; Taxi/Peter Denton 116tl; Taxi/Michael Goldman 117tr; Image Bank/Color Day Production 119br; Stone/Klaus Lahnstein 123b; Image Bank/Peter Mason 124bl; Photodisc Green 128tl; Taxi/Michael Goldman 133br; Image Bank/Tracy Frankel 141b; Photographer's Choice/Jim Bastardo 143br; Stone/Roger Charity 146bl; Thinkstock 149tr; Taxi/Antonio Mo 152; Taxi/Jim Franco 162tl; Foodpix/Burke/Triolo Productions 166b; Stone/Steve Taylor 170tl; Taxi/David Oliver 183br; Taxi/Jim Cummins 186tl; Taxi/Bill Ling 187tr; Stone/Dave Crosier 190tl; Taxi/Arthur Tilly 191tr; Image Bank/Thierry Dosogne 196tl; Stone/Elie Bernager 197tr; Stone/David Joel 207tr; Photodisc Green 172b. **SPL**: Gusto 11tr; CNRI 12bc; Astrid & Hanns-Frieder Michler 12br; BSIP, Chassenet 18tl; Faye Norman 20tl; Ruth Jenkinson/MIDIRS 20bl; Geoff Tompkinson 192bl; Custom Medical Stock Photo 193cr; Paul Parker 193br; Sue Ford 195bl; Mauro Fermariello 199br; Josh Sher 204tl; 210tl; Saturn Stills 212tl; BSIP Barrelle 213tr

All other images © Dorling Kindersley.
For further information see **www.dkimages.com**